8/24

SIRTFOOD DIET

The Ultimate Step By Step Guides To Losing Weight And Burning Fat Using The Secret Of The Famous Skinny Gene

RICHARD R. RAYMONDS

TABLE OF CONTENTS

INTRODUCTION

———— ∽ ————

W eight loss was all everyone was talking about recently, especially after pictures of singer Adele at the Oscars after-party allegedly appeared from seven stone lighter.

This comes after photos of the singer had lost three stones on a beach in Anguilla over Christmas have appeared.

How did it work out? Apparently, by taking up the Sirtfood Diet, known for actively encouraging those who observe it to get red wine and chocolate.

We can live longer sometimes, but we might not be living a healthy life.

Staggeringly, the amount of time we spent in poor health has doubled from 20 to 40 percent in a mere ten years. This means we are now spending almost 32 years of our lives in bad health. Just take a look at certain statistics. Four in ten have diabetes right now, and another three are on the verge of getting it. Two out of every five people at some stage of their lives will be diagnosed with cancer. If you see three people over fifty years old, one of them may have an osteoporotic fracture. And in the average time it takes you to read a single paragraph in this book, a new case in Alzheimer's is going to arise and someone is going to die of heart attack, and that's just in the USA.

"Dieting" was never our thing, for those reasons. That's a revolutionary modern and simple way to eat your way to weight loss and better fitness before we discovered Sirtfoods!

In recent years, the Sirtfood diet has been as common as the Cabbage Soup Diet, the 5.2 Diet, and the Dukan diet, not only popular with Adele but also with celebrities such as Lorraine Pascale and Jodie Kidd. But is it yet another diet that promises so much, or it does help you slim down and feel better adopting a sirtfood eating plan.

We talked to the experts to distinguish reality from fiction and show you what you need to know about the Sirtfood Diet.

CHAPTER ONE

WHAT IS SIRTFOODS?

Once calories are cut, this induces an energy deficit that stimulates what is known as the "skinny gene," causing a cascade of gradual change. This places the body in a sort of state of survival where fat is prevented from processing, and regular development cycles are put on hold.

Alternatively, the body concentrates its energies on burning up its fat reserves and putting them on good housekeeping genes that restore and rejuvenate our cells and give them a clean spring. The upshot is weight loss and greater resistance to disease. But cutting calories comes up at a premium, as many dietitians know. The short-term loss in energy intake induces fatigue, irritability, discomfort, and muscle weakness. Long-term limits on calories are causing slowing in our metabolism. That is the downside of all diets that are calorie-restrictive and paves the way for a piling back on the weight. Of all, 99 percent of dietitians are vulnerable to long-term deceit.

All of this has caused us to ask a big question: is it possible to activate our slim gene and all the wonderful benefits that come with all those drawbacks without having to stick to a strict calorie limit?

Enter Sirtfoods, a collection of freshly discovered wonder-foods.

Sirtfoods are especially rich in different nutrients that can cause our bodies to consume the same skinny genes that we do with calorie restriction. These proteins are termed sirtuins. They first came to light in a seminal study in 2003, when researchers discovered that resveratrol, a compound present in red grape skin and red wine, had significantly increased the yeast's lifespan. Resveratrol unbelievably had the same effect on longevity as calorie restriction, but this was achieved without increasing sugar consumption resveratrol has also been found to be capable of prolonging life in larvae, butterflies, fish, and even honeybees. Early-stage experiments from mice to humans indicate that resveratrol defends against the detrimental effects of high-calorie, high-fat, and high-sugar diets; it facilitates healthier aging by slowing down age-related diseases and increases agility; Essentially, the results of reducing calories and exercise have proven to be an imitation.

Red wine, with its rich resveratrol content, was dubbed as the first Sirtfood, describing the health advantages associated with its intake, and also why people who drink red wine get less weight. But this is just the start of the Sirtfood story.

The world of health science was at the cusp of something important with the discovery of resveratrol, and the pharmaceutical industry lost little time in getting on board. For their ability to activate our sirtuin genes, scientists started screening thousands of specific chemical compounds. This demonstrated a number of natural plant compounds with important activating properties of the sirtuin, not just resveratrol. It was also found that a given food may contain a whole range of these plant compounds which would work together to accumulate and intensify the sirtuin-activating effect of the food. It'd have been one of the most important puzzles of resveratrol. Resveratrol-experimenting scientists have needed to make a buck by delivering much greater doses than we know as part of the red wine when drunk. Nevertheless, as well as resveratrol, red wine produces many other natural compounds for plants, including large quantities of piceatannol as well as quercetin, myricetin, and epicatechin, each of which has been shown to activate our sirtuin genes independently and, more precisely, to work together.

The problem for the pharmaceutical industry is that they cannot market the next big blockbuster drug as a group of nutrients or foods. So instead, they invested hundreds of millions of dollars in the hopes of uncovering a Shangri-la pill to develop and conduct tests of synthetic compounds.

There are currently several trials of sirtuin-activating medications for a multitude of chronic disorders, as well as the first-ever FDA-approved trial to explore how a medication would delay aging.

If we've been told something from practice, it's that we shouldn't have as much appetite for this synthetic ambrosia as it may sound tantalizing. The pharmacy and wellness companies have continually sought to mimic the effects of foods and diets by extracted nutrients and medications.

And it has come up short time and again. Why wait ten more years for the legalization of these so-called miracle drugs and the unavoidable side effects they offer because we now have all the amazing benefits that we enjoy at our disposal from the food?

And since the pharmaceutical industry is actively chasing a drug like a magic bullet, our culinary focus has to be retrained. Because at the same time, those efforts were underway, the nutritional research landscape was also shifting, raising some of its big questions. Red wine on one side, were there other high-level foods of these special nutrients able to activate our sirtuin genes? And if so, what effects did they have on causing weight loss and preventing disease?

Not All Fruits And Vegetables Are Created Equal

Researchers at Harvard University have performed two of the largest medical surveys in U.S. history since 1986: the Health Practitioners Follow-Up Study, which explores men's eating patterns and wellbeing, and the Nurses' Wellness Report, which discusses the same for mothers. Based on this overwhelming wealth of evidence, researchers investigated the link between the dietary patterns of over 124,000 people and improvements in body weight over 24 years ended in 2011

They noticed it interesting. Consuming other plant foods stayed off weight gain as part of a typical American diet, but eating others did not affect whatsoever. What was their difference? It all boiled down to whether there were other forms of natural plant chemicals such as polyphenols that made the food rich. Almost all of us continue to weigh as we grow, but eating higher concentrations of polyphenols was extraordinary.

Effect of keeping this from occurring. Only some forms of polyphenols stand out when tested in greater depth as being effective in keeping people thin, the researchers found.

And these were the same classes of natural plant chemicals that the pharmaceutical industry was desperately attempting to turn into a miracle pill because of their potential to turn our sirtuin genes on.

The conclusion was profound: When it comes to controlling our weight, not all plant foods (including fruits and vegetables) are equal. Instead, we need to start researching plant foods for their polyphenol content and then investigate their ability to switch on our "skinny" sirtuin genes.

This is a radical idea that runs counter to our time's prevailing dogma. It's time to let go of the conventional blanket recommendation that asks us to eat as part of a healthy diet two cups of fruit and two and a half cups of vegetables a day. We just need to look around to see how little it has had effects.

Everything more became evident with this change in deciding whether plant foods are healthy for us. The many foods that supposedly health experts cautioned us about, such as chocolate, coffee, and tea, are so abundant in sirtuin-activating polyphenols that they beat most fruits and vegetables out there. So many times, are we grimacing as we chew our veggies when we are told that this is the best thing to do, just to feel bad should we even look at the candy cookie after dinner? The biggest irony is that cacao is one of the greatest things that we could be consuming. Its intake has now been shown to activate sirtuin genes, with several benefits for regulating body weight by consuming fat, decreasing appetite, and increasing muscle function. So this is when we take the plethora of other health advantages into account, more of which will come later.

In total, we have identified foods rich in polyphenols that have been shown to activate our sirtuin genes, and together these form the basis of the Sirtfood Diet. While the tale started as the original Sirtfood with red wine, we now know that these other nineteen foods equal or beat it for their sirtuin-activating polyphenol content. In addition to cocoa, these include other well-known and enjoyable foods such as extra virgin olive oil, red onions, garlic, parsley, chilies, kale, strawberries, walnuts, capers, tofu, green tea, and even coffee. Although each food has amazing health credentials of its own, as we are about to see, when we mix these foods to make a whole diet, the real magic happens.

A Common Link Among The World's Healthiest Diets

When we further researched, we discovered that the best concentrations of sirtfoods were found in the diets of those with the lowest disease and obesity levels in the world — from the Kuna American Indians, who are resistant to high blood pressure and exhibit surprisingly low levels of hypertension, diabetes, cancer, and early death, thanks to a fantastically rich consumption of Sirtfood cocoa; to Okinawa, Japan,

But it's the lifestyle that is the envy of the rest of the Western world, a conventional Mediterranean lifestyle, where Sirtfoods especially stands out for its benefits. Obesity does not exist here, and the difference is a medical disease, not the rule. Extra virgin olive oil, wild leafy vegetables, almonds, fruit, red wine, dates, and herbs are also strong syrups, and appearing prominently in Mediterranean native diets. Given the new opinion that adopting a Mediterranean diet is more effective than counting calories for weight loss, and more effective than prescription medications to combat the disease, the scientific community has been left in awe.

This brings us to the 2013 publication of PREDIMED, a game-changing study of the Mediterranean Diet. It was tested on about 7,400 people at high risk of cardiovascular disease, and the findings were so positive that the study was practically ended early — after only five years. PREDIMED's idea was gorgeously plain. This asked what the difference between a Mediterranean-style diet supplemented by either extra virgin olive oil or nuts (especially walnuts) and a more traditional modern-day diet would be. And what a difference.

The dietary adjustment reduced the incidence of cardiovascular disease by around 30 percent, and drug makers can only think of a return. Following further follow-up, a 30 percent drop in diabetes was also found, along with significant drops in inflammation, improvements in memory and brain health, and a massive 40 percent reduction in obesity, with significant fat loss, especially around the stomach area.

But researchers were initially unable to clarify what these drastic benefits were. Neither the quantities of calories, fats, and sugars eaten — the usual tests used to determine the food we eat — nor the rate of physical exercise separated within the classes to illustrate the findings. Anything still has to get moving.

The eureka moment then happened. Both extra virgin olive oil and walnuts stand out for their exceptional content of polyphenols, which activate sirtuin. Essentially, by adding these to a standard Mediterranean diet in large quantities, what the researchers unwittingly produced was a super-rich Sirtfood diet, and they found it delivered incredible results.

But PREDIMED-analyzing researchers came up with a smart idea. If essentially it is the polyphenols that count, they mused, perhaps those who eat more of them would reap their combined benefits by living the longest. So they were running the statistics, and the results were staggering. Those who consumed the highest polyphenol levels had 37 percent fewer deaths over just five years compared to those who ate the least.

Intriguingly, this is double the reduction in mortality, which is found to bring in treatment with the most commonly prescribed blockbuster statin drugs. Finally, we had the reason for the mind-blowing benefits found in this test, and it was more effective than any current medication.

The researchers also noticed anything else interesting. While previously, many studies have found that individual Sirtfoods confer impressive health benefits; they have never been deep enough to extend life. The first one was the PREDIMED. The difference was that they were looking at a food pattern rather than a single food. Different foods provide different polyphenols that activate sirtuin, which work in harmony to produce a much more powerful result than any single food can. It has left an irrepressible impression for us. True health is not caught by a single nutrient or even a "wonder food." What you need is a complete diet with a combination of synergistic Sirtfoods. And that is what led to Sirtfood Diet being developed.

Is Sirtfoods the New Superfoods?

There's no doubt that Sirtfoods is the best for you. They also have a high nutrient content and are made of good plant compounds.

Besides, studies have associated health benefits to many of the foods recommended on the Sirtfood Diet.

Eating moderate quantities of dark chocolate with a high content of cacao, for example, can reduce the risk of heart disease and help fight inflammation.

Drinking green tea will decrease the risk of stroke and diabetes and rising blood pressure.

And turmeric has anti-inflammatory properties that usually have positive effects on the body, and can also guard against chronic inflammatory diseases.

Most sirtfoods have reportedly shown health benefits in humans.

Data on the health effects of increasing the levels of sirtuin protein is tentative, however. Yet animal and cell line research have been showing exciting results.

Researchers have found, for example, that increased levels of some sirtuin proteins lead to a longer lifespan in yeast, worms, and mice.

And the sirtuin proteins instruct the body to consume more fat for energy and increase insulin sensitivity during fasting or calorie restriction. One mice study found that increased levels of sirtuin led to a loss of fat.

Any research indicates sirtuins may also play a role in reducing inflammation, inhibiting tumor growth, and delaying heart disease and Alzheimer's growth.

While studies have shown positive results in mice and human cell lines, no human studies have examined the effects of increasing sirtuin levels.

Therefore it is unclear whether elevated levels of sirtuin protein in the body would lead to longer lifetime or lower risk of human cancer.

New work is underway to produce compounds that are effective at rising sirtuin levels in the body. It helps clinical research to continue investigating the impact of sirtuins on human wellbeing.

Safety and side effects

While the Sirtfood Diet's first phase is very low in calories and nutritionally incomplete, there are no real safety concerns for the average, healthy adult considering the short duration of the diet. Yet for someone with diabetes, reducing calories and only consuming juice for the first few days of the diet may cause harmful changes in blood sugar levels.

Nevertheless, even a healthy person can suffer certain side effects — primarily hunger.

Eating just 1,000–1,500 calories per day will leave just about anyone feeling hungry, especially if much of what you're eating is a juice that's low in fiber, a nutrient that helps you stay full.

During phase one, due to the calorie restriction, you might experience other side effects such as fatigue, lightheadedness, and irritability.

Serious health consequences are rare for a stable adult, provided the diet is followed.

CHAPTER TWO

THE SCIENCE OF SIRTUINS

Wat makes the Sirtfood Diet so strong is their capacity to turn to an ancient gene family that resides within each of us. The name for the gene family is sirtuin. Sirtuins are different as they orchestrate mechanisms deep inside our cells that include issues as important as our capacity to lose fat, our resistance to disease or not, and eventually also our life span. The influence of sirtuins is so significant that they are now referred to as "chief metabolic regulators." Basically, what exactly someone who wishes to lose a few pounds and lead a long and happy life will like to be in control of.

Of Mice And Men

In recent years, sirtuins have become understandably, the subject of intense scientific research. The first sirtuin was detected in yeast back in 1984, and research really began over the course of the next three decades when it was revealed that sirtuin activation enhances life span, first in yeast and then all the way up to mice.

Why the thrills? Since the fundamental rules of cellular metabolism are nearly similar from yeast to humans, and all in between. If you can control anything as small as a burgeoning yeast and see a benefit, then replicate it in higher species like mice, there is hope for the same benefits to be discovered in humans.

An appetite for fasting?

Which brings us to fasting. Consistently, the lifetime reduction of food consumption has been found to increase the life span of lower species and mammals. This extraordinary discovery is the basis for the custom of caloric restriction by certain individuals, where daily calorie consumption is lowered by about 20 to 30 per cent, as well as its popularized offshoot, intermittent fasting, which has become a common weight-loss diet, made famous by the likes of the 5:2 diet, or Easy Diet. Although we are still seeking proof of improved longevity for humans from these activities, there is proof of improvements of what we could term "health span"—chronic sickness decreases, and obesity starts of melt away.

But let's be honest, no matter how huge the advantages, fasting week in, week out, is a grueling enterprise that most of us don't want to sign up for. Even if we do, most of us are not able to stick to this.

Besides this there are risks to fasting, particularly if we practice it for a long time. We listed in the introduction the side effects of hunger, irritability, weakness, muscle failure and slowing in metabolism. Yet current fasting programs may also place us at risk of starvation, impacting our well-being due to a decreased intake of vital nutrients. Fasting regimens are therefore entirely inadequate for significant numbers of the

Population such as infants, pregnant women and, most likely, elderly people. Although fasting has obviously proven advantages, it's not the silver bullet we 'd want it to be. It had us ask, is this really the way Nature was meant to make us thin and healthy? There's definitely a safer way out there.

Our breakthrough came when we discovered that our ancient

sirtuin genes were activated by mediating the profound benefits from caloric restriction and fasting. Thinking of sirtuins as the guardians at the crossroads of energy status and immortality may be helpful to better understand this. There, what they do is react to stresses.

When energy is in short supply, there is an rise in tension on our cells just as we see in the calorie limit. The sirtuins sensed this, which then switched on and transmitted a constellation of powerful signals that radically altered the behavior of cells. Sirtuins boost our metabolism, increase muscle capacity, turn on fat burning, decrease inflammation and repair any cell damage. In turn, the sirtuins make us more fit, more lean and more safe.

Sirtfoods Versus Fasting

This leads to a big question: if activation of the sirtuin increases muscle mass, why do we lose muscle when we fast? Fasting also stimulates our sirtuin genes.

Bear with us as we dig through the mechanics of this. Not all skeletal muscles are created equal to each other. We have two main types, named type-1 and type-2, conveniently. Type-1 muscle is used for movements of longer duration, while the type-2 muscle is used for short bursts of more intense activity. And here it gets intriguing: Fasting only increases SIRT1 activity in muscle fibers type-1, not type-2. The thickness of the muscle fiber type-1 is thus preserved, and even when we strong, it increases noticeably. Sadly, incomplete comparison to what occurs during fasting in type-1 fibers, SIRT1 decreases quickly in type-2 fibers. This means the fat-burning slows down, and muscle breaks down to provide heat, instead.

So fasting for the muscles is a double-edged sword, with our type-2 fibers taking a hit. Type-2 fibers form the majority of our concept of muscle. And even though our type-1 fiber mass is growing fast, we also see a substantial total loss of muscle. If we were able to avoid the breakdown, it would not only make us look aesthetically healthy but also encourage more weight loss. So the way to achieve so is to combat the decrease in SIRT1 in muscle fiber type-2 that is caused by fasting.

Scientists at Harvard Medical School tested this in an elegant mice trial and found that the signals for muscle breakdown were turned off by inducing SIRT1 activity in type-2 fibers during fasting, and no muscle damage occurred.

The researchers then went a step further and tested the effects of increased SIRT1 activity on the muscle while the mice were fed rather than fasted, and found it caused a very rapid growth of the muscle. Within a week, muscle fibers with elevated levels of SIRT1 activity displayed an impressive weight gain of 20 percent.

Such results are somewhat close to the outcome of our Sirtfood Diet experiment, but in turn, our research has been milder. Through increasing SIRT1 activity and consuming a diet rich in sirtfoods, most participants had no muscle loss — and for others, it was just a mild strength, muscle mass that increased.

Fighting fat.

Some of the surprising results from our Sirtfood Diet pilot study wasn't just how much weight the participants lost, which was amazing enough — it was the amount of weight loss that most fascinated us. What caught our attention was the fact that a lot of people lost weight without losing any muscle. Seeing people gain muscle wasn't uncommon.

This left us with an unavoidable conclusion: fat had merely melted away.

Achieving a substantial fat reduction usually involves a tremendous effort, either significantly restricting calories or participating in extraordinary workout levels. Yet counter to this, our participants either retained or reduced their rates of exercise, and did not even mention feeling particularly hungry. In reality, some even failed to consume all of the food they had been supplied with.

How much is that possible? Only when we realize what happens to our fat cells when there is elevated sirtuin production can we begin to make sense of these amazing findings.

Appetite control.

There was one thing we couldn't get our minds around in our pilot study: the people didn't necessarily get hungry, given a drop in calories. In reality, some people struggled to consume all of the food that was offered.

One of the major advantages of the Sirtfood Diet is that without the need for a long-term calorie limit, we can reap great benefits. The very first week of diet is the process of hyper-success, where we pair mild fasting with an excess of strong Sirtfoods for a double blow to weight. And we predicted any signs of hunger here, as with all of the fasting regimens. Yet we've had absolutely zero!

We sought the solution as we trawled through analysis. It's all thanks to the body's main appetite-regulating hormone, leptin, called the "satiety hormone." As we feed, leptin decreases, signaling the hypothalamus inhibiting desire to a section of the brain. Conversely, leptin signaling to the brain declines as we fly, which makes us feel hungry.

Leptin is so effective in controlling appetite that early expectations could be used as a "silver bullet" for combating obesity. But that dream was shattered by the realization that the metabolic dysfunction occurring in obesity causes leptin to stop properly working. In obesity, the amount of leptin that can enter the brain decreases, but the hypothalamus is often desensitized to its behavior. That's it

Known as leptin resistance: leptin is present but doesn't work properly anymore. Thus, with certain overweight people, the brain tends to believe they are underfed even though they consume plenty, which signals for them to try to pursue calories.

The consequence of this is that while the amount of leptin in the blood is necessary to control appetite, how much of it enters the brain and its effect on the hypothalamus is much more relevant. It is here that the Sirtfoods shine.

New research demonstrates that the nutrients present in Sirtfoods have important advantages in overcoming leptin resistance. This is by both increasing leptin transport to the brain and increasing the hypothalamus' sensitivity to leptin actions.

So back to our original question: Why don't the Sirtfood Diet make people feel hungry? Given a decrease in blood leptin levels during the mild quick, which would usually increase hunger, adding Sirtfoods into the diet makes leptin signals more effective, leading to better control of appetite.

As we'll see later, Sirtfoods also has strong effects on our taste centers, ensuring we get a lot more enjoyment and gratification from our food and thus don't slip into the overeating pit to feel good.

Sirtuins are expected to be a brand new term for only the most committed dietitians. But hitting the sirtuins, our metabolism 's master regulators, is the foundation of every effective diet for weight loss. Tragically, the very nature of our modern society, with abundant food and sedentary lifestyles, creates a perfect storm to shut down our sirtuin activity. We see all around us the consequences of this.

The good news is that we now know what sirtuins are, how fat accumulation is managed, and how fat burning is encouraged, and, most importantly, how to turn them on. And with this revolutionary breakthrough, the answer to effective and sustained weight loss is ultimately yours to take.

A zeal for exercise?

It's not just calorie limitation and fasting that stimulates sirtuins; exercise always does. As in fasting, sirtuins orchestrate is the fundamental benefits of exercise. Even while we are urged to participate in routine, moderate exercise for its multitude of advantages, it is not the means on which we are expected to concentrate our attention on weight-loss. Evidence indicates that the human body has developed ways of adapting spontaneously and that the amount of energy that we expend while exercising, which ensures that in order for exercise to be a successful weight-loss strategy, we need to devote considerable time and effort.

That grueling fitness regimens is the way nature designed us to sustain a healthier weight is much more questionable in the light of studies now showing that too much fitness may be harmful weakening our immune systems, damaging the heart and leading to early death.

Enter Sirtfoods

So far we have discovered that the key to activating our sirtuin genes is if we want to lose weight and be healthy. Fasting and exercise have been the two known ways of doing that up to now.

Unfortunately, the quantities needed for good weight loss come with their pitfalls, and for most of us, this is clearly inconsistent with how we lead twenty-first century lives. Thankfully, there is a recently found, ground-breaking way to activate our sirtuin genes in the best way possible: sirtfood. As we will learn in the near future, these are the wonder foods that are particularly rich in special natural plant chemicals that have the potential to talk to and switch on our sirtuin genes. In reality, they mimic the results of fasting and exercise and thus deliver remarkable previously unattainable benefits of weight loss , muscle building and health enhancement.

CHAPTER THREE

WELL-BEING WONDERS

Society is getting fatter and sicker given all the impressive developments in medical medicine—70 percent of all deaths are attributed to infectious illness, a profoundly startling figure. Extreme, and fast, reform is required.

Yet as we've learned, all of that will continue to shift. We will burn fat by triggering our ancient sirtuin genes and create a leaner, stronger body. And with sirtuins at the center of our metabolism, our biology master programmers, their importance reaches well beyond the structure of the body itself, to every aspect of our well-being.

Sirtuins and the 70 percent.

Think of a disease you equate with getting old, and the odds are that there is a lack of sirtuin production involved in the body. For example, sirtuin activation is excellent for the heart muscle protection, strengthening the heart muscle cells and simply improving the heart muscle function. This also strengthens the way our arteries function, allows them to treat cholesterol more efficiently and saves us from the blockage in our arteries known as atherosclerosis.

As with diabetes? Sirtuin activation increases the amount of insulin that can be secreted and makes the body more effective. When it occurs, metformin, one of the most commonly used antidiabetic medications, depends on SIRT1 for its beneficial function.

Indeed, one pharmaceutical firm is actively exploring natural sirtuin activators' application to diabetic metformin therapy, with findings from animal trials showing a remarkable 83% reduction in the metformin dose needed for the same impact.

As for the brain, sirtuins are also active, with sirtuin expression lower in patients with Alzheimer's. By comparison, stimulation of the sirtuin increases feedback patterns in the brain, promotes executive performance, and decreases inflammation in the brain. It prevents the buildup of amyloid-β production and tau protein aggregation, two of the most detrimental factors we find occurring in the brains of people with Alzheimer's.

The next one is the bones. Osteoblasts are a special type of cell that is responsible for creating new bone in our bodies. The more osteoblasts we get, the healthier our bones are. Sirtuin activation not only facilitates osteoblast cell growth but also enhances its survival. This makes activation of the sirtuin central to lifelong bone safety.

For sirtuin science, cancer has become a more contentious area. Although recent work suggests that sirtuin activation helps suppress cancer tumors, scientists are just beginning to unravel this complicated region. While there is much more to learn about this particular issue, as we shall see soon, the lowest cancer levels are seen in those communities that consume the most Sirtfoods.

Heart disease, arthritis, dementia, osteoporosis, and most likely cancer: there is a remarkable list of diseases that can be avoided by sirtuin activation. It can be no surprise that communities now consume lots of Sirtfoods as part of their conventional diets can hardly envision a resilience and well-being that you'll learn more about very soon.

This leaves us with an interesting conclusion: simply by introducing the most strong sirtfoods in the world to your diet and making it a lifetime routine, you too will achieve this level of well-being — and more — when you get the science you like.

Sirtfoods.

We've learned so far that sirtuins are an ancient gene family with the ability to help us lose weight, create muscle, and keep us super healthy. It is well known that through dietary limitation, fasting, and exercise, sirtuins can be turned on, but there is another innovative way to do this: diet. We refer to the most potent foods to activate sirtuins as Sirtfoods.

Beyond antioxidants.

To better appreciate the benefits of Sirtfoods, we need to learn about foods like fruits and vegetables very differently, and why they are perfect for us. Despite tons of evidence demonstrating that diets high in fruits, vegetables, and processed products usually cut the risk of multiple infectious illnesses, including the greatest killers, heart failure, and cancer, there is no denying that they do. It has been put down to their rich nutritional content, such as vitamins, minerals, and antioxidants, which is perhaps the best wellness buzzword of the past decade. Yet this is a very different story we are here to share.

The explanation Sirtfoods is so amazing for you has nothing to do with the nutrients that we all know so well and hear about so much. Yes, they're all important items you need to get out of your diet, but with Sirtfoods, there's something completely different, and very rare. What if we threw the entire way of thought on its head and said that the reason Sirtfoods is good for you is not that they nourish the body with vital nutrients, or have antioxidants to mop up the damaging effects of free radicals, but quite the opposite: because they are full of weak toxins? This could sound insane in a world where almost every alleged "superfood" is actively promoted based on its antioxidant content. But it's a groundbreaking concept, and one worth taking on.

What doesn't kill you makes you stronger

Let's go back for a moment to the proven methods of activating sirtuins: fasting and exercise. Evidence has demonstrated consistently, as we have shown, that the allocation of dietary resources has significant effects on weight loss, well-being, and, quite likely, lifespan. There is fitness, borne out by the discovery that daily exercise significantly slashes death rates and has endless advantages for both body and mind. But what is it they have in common?

The solution lies in: heat. Both fasting and exercise allow the body to experience moderate stress, which helps it adapt by being stronger, more productive, and more resilient. The reaction of the body to such slightly unpleasant stimuli — its adaptation — that, in the long run, should make us happier, safer, and leaner. And as we now know, sirtuins orchestrate these extremely beneficial adaptations, which are turned on in the presence of these stressors, and spark a host of desirable changes in the body.

The scientific word used to respond to such stresses is hormesis. It's the principle that if subjected to a small dosage of a drug or stimulus that is either harmful or deadly, if administered at higher doses, you get a beneficial result. Or "what doesn't kill you makes you stronger," if you choose. And that's exactly how fasting and exercise work. Hunger is fatal, so regular exercise is prejudicial to safety.

Enter Polyphenols

Now, here's when things get interesting. Both living species undergo hormesis, but the fact that this even involves plants is what has been highly undervalued until now.

While we would not usually think of plants as being the same as other living species, let alone humans, we do share common responses in terms of how we respond to our environment on a chemical basis.

As mind-blowing as that sounds, it makes perfect sense to think evolutionarily about it, because all living things have evolved to cope with common environmental stresses such as dehydration, sunlight, deprivation of nutrients, and Pathogens kill.

If that's hard to wrap your head around, get ready for the genuinely awesome part. Reactions to plant tension are, in general, more complex than ours. Think about it: if we are starving and thirsty, we can go looking for food and drink; too dry, we need shade; we can see under attack. In full comparison, plants are stagnant, and as such, all the severity of these physiological pressures and challenges must survive. As a result, they have built a highly complex stress-response mechanism over the past billion years that humble everything we can boast about. The way they do this is to create a huge array of natural plant chemicals — called polyphenols — that will help them to adapt to their climate and thrive. We also absorb certain polyphenol nutrients when we eat these plants. Their influence is profound: they activate our inherent mechanisms to react to stress. There we are thinking about almost the same pathways that turn on to fasting and exercise: the sirtuins.

Piggybacking on the stress-response mechanism of a plant in this way is known as xenohormesis for our benefit. And the effects of this are game-changing. Let the plants do the hard work, and we do not. Indeed, because of their potential to toggle on the same beneficial improvements in our bodies, such as fat burning, as can be seen during fasting, these natural plant compounds are often referred to as caloric restricting mimetics. By supplying us with more sophisticated signaling compounds than we are generating ourselves, they cause effects comparable to anything that can be obtained by eating or exercising alone.

Sirtfoods around the world

Sirtfoods may be a new culinary innovation, but it's obvious that throughout history, diverse societies have enjoyed their benefits. As we are more acquainted with the top twenty Sirtfoods in chapter below, we can see how many have been valued for their medicinal properties since early history, and have also been considered sacred foods for their ability to impart vigor and well-being.

Yes, it now seems that published evidence of these Sirtfoods benefits goes back a long way to being the subject of the very first clinical trial ever conducted. He was documented in the Book of Daniel in the Bible more than 2,200 years ago, we and him. It was considered the best food possible of the day and was recommended to keep the young people alive and eventually join the monarch's service. And, when Daniel opposed this, a plant-only diet yielded a better outcome in only a couple of days: "Daniel made up his mind not to let himself become ritually unclean by consuming the rich food and drinking the royal court's wine. Daniel went to the guard, then. He said, check us out for ten days. Bring us [plant] vegetables to feed and drink tea. Compare us with the young men who eat the royal court's food and base your opinion on how we feel. He decided to give them ten days to check it out. When the time was up, it was found that in presentation, they were stronger and fatter in fresh [muscular] than all who had eaten the royal meal. And the guard should let them keep eating vegetables instead of what the king received.

Such benefits should usually never be expected from a diet of only plants, particularly increased muscle mass. This, of course, is because certain plants were incredibly rich sources of Sirtfood. With reports revealing that the typical plants eaten back then were identical to the Sirtfood-rich conventional Mediterranean diet, and findings remarkably close to our pilot experiment, one can't help wonder whether the Daniel study is the stuff of fable, or do we unwittingly have the solution to achieving the body and well-being we've all desired for over two millennia?

Enter The Blue Zone

Though our health is ailing, there are areas worldwide, called Blue Zones, where Sirtfoods consumption is much higher than the amount we eat in a standard Western diet.

Indeed, the effects sound more like the stuff of myth to communities eating Sirtfood-rich diets. In fact, not only do we see people live longer in Blue Zones than in countries where a traditional Western diet is a norm, but the way they maintain youthful stamina in old age is even more significant. In the Blue Areas, the levels of Alzheimer's, cancer, diabetes, lung disease, and osteoporosis are extremely low. Go there, and you will see people aged 90 or older walking, laughing, and working. We are not involved in the promotion of weight loss; there is no need for a gym. Alternatively, young people maintain their vigor and vitality until old age. You'll see them in the street on motorbikes or ride bicycles. Have a conversation with them, and you might hear them bragging how wonderful their sex life is now! And it's no joke they do happen to be the world's slimmest people.

I Should Cocoa

To fully understand this amazing trend, let's continue our adventure with a trip for Panama's San Blas Islands, the Kuna American Indians' ancestral home, which is immune to high blood pressure and displays surprisingly low levels of hypertension, diabetes, cancer and early death. A work team discovered the origin of the Kuna at the turn of the twenty-first century when they found out their primary source of liquid was a beverage made from local cocoa. This cocoa is fantastic in a particular group of polyphenols called flavanols, particularly epicatechin, characterizing it as syrtfood.

But how do we learn that the Kuna's robust well-being was due to their strong cocoa flavanol intake? The researchers found that the health benefits ended as the Kuna Indians moved to Panama City and shifted to drinking intensively refined commercial cocoa (which is deprived of its flavanols and thus no longer a Sirtfood).

The Kuna case is just one piece of growing evidence that flavanol-rich cocoa has exceptional benefits for health. Clinical trials have found flavanol-rich cocoa to boost blood pressure, blood supply, blood sugar regulation, and cholesterol levels.

Reviews say cocoa has positive effects on diabetes and cancer as well. Consumption has been shown to boost memory capacity and to have a Dietary beneficial choice in Youth Fountain Brain.

So despite the repeated reminders that chocolate is bad for you, we now know that cacao improves oral hygiene, so it protects the teeth from plaque and cavities.

Spice For Life

For more than 4,000 years, Turmeric, known as "Indian solid gold," has been used for wound healing and anti-inflammatory effects in Ayurvedic medicine. We now realize that these calming properties are because it contains curcumin, a significant nutrient that stimulates sirtuin, rendering it a syrtfood.

Turmeric is a prevalent spice in conventional Indian cuisine and is suspected of leading to slightly lower cancer rates in India than in Western countries. Interestingly, however, as they switch from India to the US or UK and leave their conventional diet, the cancer risk for Indians rises by 50 to 75 percent. Although this may be attributed to a variety of various influences in the diet, experimental research now indicates that curcumin has strong anticancer properties.

Aside from its claims to be anticancer, there is mounting evidence of other health benefits that activate sirtuin. In recent years, it has been shown that a special form of curcumin that has been designed to digest more quickly has increased cholesterol levels, enhanced blood sugar regulation, and decreased body inflammation. It was tested for knee osteoarthritis and found to be as successful as painkillers usually used. Researchers are now exposing their multiple strategies to discourage weight gain and to help combat obesity. And in people with early type 2 diabetes, their working memory strengthened by eating only one gram of Turmeric a day.

Green Living

Green tea is another beguiling deal from Sirtfood. Green tea use is believed to have begun more than 4,700 years ago when, through serendipity, the Chinese emperor Shen Nung ("Divine Healer") made a delicious, soothing drink with green tea leaves. And much later did the product establish its reputation for medical strength and healing.

Asia 's high green tea consumption has been cited as a primary explanation for the "Asian paradox." Given the extremely high prevalence of cigarette smoking, Asia and particularly Japan boasts some of the lowest coronary disease and lung cancer rates in the world. High consumption of green tea is associated with slightly lower levels of coronary heart disease and a lowered incidence of certain cancers, such as prostate, liver, lung, and breast. Therefore it is no surprise that green tea use is related to slightly less early deaths.

Green tea also has a thermogenic effect, meaning it raises the number of calories the body burns down and helps lose weight while maintaining muscle. Combine green tea with an abundant diet of leafy greens, soybeans, herbs, and spices (turmeric usage is especially prevalent) to create a meal of syrtle foods. We have a diet very close to that found in Okinawa—"the land of the immortals. "Okinawa may be the poorest province in Japan, but it has historical longevity and the highest number of centenarians in the world. Their quality of life is so incredible, and researchers thought it must be attributed to superior genes. But the Westernization of the diet came along and with it burgeoning levels of obesity and debilitating diseases that younger generations are now encountering for the first time, putting firmly to rest the notion of superior biology.

A Mediterranean Prescription

We need to fly to the Mediterranean for a real abundance of the Sirtfood varieties. This is where we come together with a host of potent Sirtfoods, including extra virgin olive oil, almonds, fruits, green leafy vegetables, herbs and spices, and wine. Eating this type of diet is associated with a 9 percent reduction in all-cause mortality, with substantial reductions in cardiovascular disease and degenerative brain diseases such as Alzheimer's and cancer. And as we saw in our review, the seminal PREDIMED trial in Spain found that the occurrence of cardiovascular disease and diabetes was cut by a Mediterranean-style diet supplemented with either extra virgin olive oil or nuts (especially walnuts)

In the PREDIMED sub-sample, researchers even did something really important. They looked at the genetic profile for PPAR-ÿ — which, as you recall, is the obesity antagonist we've found before. Although some of us are very immune to their acts, some are not so lucky, and can get clobbered by them. It suggests that you can eat the same as anyone else but maybe far more vulnerable to adding weight. It doesn't need to be like that with Sirtfoods, though. The negative effects of this gene have been reversed in those who adopted the Sirtfood-rich Mediterranean diet. Incredibly, the diet richer in Sirtfoods, despite no drop in calories, was linked to a 40 percent drop in the risk of obesity, particularly weight stored around the tummy. Forget low fat, and forget obsessed about calories: anyone adopting a conventional Mediterranean diet will still be slimmer than the general population.

And there we have it. There is much in common with communities around the world whose leaders are healthiest and slimmest and who lead the longest lives: they eat the largest quantity of syrtfood. We stay slender and lean, without counting a calorie or being on a diet. That leaves us to do only one thing: pull together all the best syrtfoods on the planet to produce a diet that has never been seen before — in reality, a diet to fuel a health and weight loss revolution.

CHAPTER FOUR

WHAT DIETITIANS REALLY THINK OF THE SIRTFOOD DIET

Earlier, after Adele's pictures appeared significantly slimmer, eyes quickly switched on how the star lost a whopping seven stone. Reports indicated that the impetus behind the Sirtfood Diet was Aidan Goggins and Glen Matten, who both hold master degrees in nutritional medicine. Adele 's former personal trainer Camila Goodis said during a January TV interview that she thought Adele was working out, but the diet was down to 90% of her weight loss.

The Sirtfood Diet is a metabolism-enhancing system that lets you drink red wine and coffee, and eat candy, which sounds like a fantasy. Yet we all know that there's no such thing as a golden weight-loss bullet, so we asked dietitians Sophie Medlin from City Dietitians and Lola Biggs, the dietitian supplement company Together Health to do some work on all sirtfood kinds of stuff.

The writers of the Sirtfood Diet say it's a way to move weight without significantly dieting as it stimulates the same receptors of the 'skinny gene' normally caused by fasting and exercise. "These foods contain chemicals called polyphenols that exert mild stress on our cells, leading to genes that mimic the fasting and exercise results. Foods rich in polyphenols these as broccoli, dark chocolate, and red wine activate sirtuin receptors that affect appetite, aging, and mood.

Research promoting the notion of foods like chili and green tea for weight loss and red wine (rich in polyphenols) is frequently quoted in the French paradox, which is why French people drink red wine but stay slim. However, there is no scientific proof to date that we can rely on that the sirtfood hypothesis is working.

The Sirtfood diet was known as the "alternative to traditional diets," according to Goggins. He and his partner, Glen Matten, were both "nutrition skeptics," because of their experience as natural health experts. The Sirtfood diet focuses on activating the sirtuin genes instead of focusing on weight reduction.

"The decrease of weight is not the primary objective, but as part of the biochemical rejuvenation of our cell well-being, which slowly resets our metabolism," Goggins said. "In comparison, unlike certain conventional diets that focus on cutting goods, we can only enjoy the advantages of consuming Sirtfoods, which means indulging in your favorite foods and not limiting them."

Kirkpatrick, who works with Cleveland Clinic in Ohio, said she had patients coming several times to ask her about the Sirtfood diet. While there is some evidence to support its results, she said all of the research and observations are very new.

"I think the diet is healthy because we don't have any evidence to show it's longevity in the long run," she said. "The entire premise behind the diet is that certain foods will induce certain sirtuins which are related to the body's proteins."

Kirkpatrick noted that the Sirtfood diet operates similarly to intermittent fasting diets that were also shown to help with weight loss.

Goggins said they were "increasingly obsessed" about "increasingly unhealthy food habits," and people were "villainizing" products while he and Matten trained at the London high-end private fitness club.

"Sugar will terrify you," he said. "And all of that was about calorie consumption cuts."

They needed to ensure that people were able to consume more of their preferred foods to have essential nutrients as they shaped their diet.

"It's important that we not only have enough of these foods in our diet but also make sure that our meals contain a number of them because they're the mixture of their meal and juice from which the real benefits come," Googins said.

A nutritionist 's final thoughts on the Sirtfood Diet

Michele says it's no surprise people will see a rapid weight loss if they reduce their calorie intake, especially during the first week of the diet. Still, she says she's very careful about encouraging people to count calories.

Nonetheless, she sees a big advantage in growing your dietary intake based on sirtuin, saying that any diet high in whole foods without adding sugars will improve your Health.

"Sirtfoods induce fat burning but also facilitate muscle growth, regeneration, and repair. Eating foods that are naturally abundant in sirtuin activators as an alternative to polyphenol supplements could be healthier, more efficient – and cheaper, "she added.

Yeah, you got it. While the Sirtfood diet has the right idea to promote the rise in whole food we can eat, the calorie counting motivation isn't exactly the healthiest path you might take on your well-being journey.

This is also a huge step towards a healthy, more appropriate lifestyle to focus on keeping a balanced, sirt-rich diet and adding physical fitness into the daytime.

CHAPTER FIVE

HOW THE SIRTFOOD DIET WILL WORK FOR YOU

The sheer range of benefits enjoyed by people has been a surprise, all done by merely basing their diet on available and inexpensive foods that most people already enjoy consuming. And this is all that the Sirtfood Diet requires. It's about extracting the advantages of daily foods that we've all been used to consume, but in the right proportions and formulations to give us the body structure and health we need

Everybody desires something very desperately, and that will fundamentally change our lives.

It doesn't require you to execute extreme calorie restrictions, nor does it require grueling exercise regimens (although staying consistently active is a good thing, of course). And just a juicer is the only piece of equipment you'll require. Plus, unlike any other diet out there that focuses on what to eliminate, the Sirtfood Diet focuses on what to add.

How to follow the Sirtfood diet.

The Sirtfood Diet has two phases that last three weeks altogether. You will then "sirtify" your diet by adding as many sirtfoods as possible into your meals.

The basic recipes for these two phases can be found in the book The Sirtfood Diet, which was published by makers of the diet. You'll need to do something to keep up with the diet.

The meals are full of sirtfoods but in addition to the "top 20 sirtfoods," other ingredients do.

Most sirtfoods and ingredients are easy to find.

Three of the signature ingredients required for these two phases, matcha green tea powder, lovage, and buckwheat — may be costly or hard to find.

A big part of the diet is the green tea, which you'll have to make between one and three times a day. A juicer (a blender won't work) and a kitchen scale will be needed, as the ingredients are listed by weight.

Phase 1

Welcome to Sirtfood Diet, phase 1. This is the process of hyper-success, where you will take a huge step towards achieving a slimmer, leaner body. Follow our simple step-by-step instructions and use the tasty recipes you'll get. We do have a meat-free option in addition to our regular seven-day program, which is ideal for vegetarians and vegans alike. Feel free to go ahead with whatever you want.

What to expect.

You'll reap the full benefits of our clinically proven method of losing 7 pounds in seven days during Phase 1. But note that involves adding weight, so don't hang up simply on the numbers on the scales. Nor should you get used to measuring yourself every day. Besides, in the last few days of Phase 1, we always see the scales rising due to muscle growth, while waistlines tend to shrink. Therefore we want you to look at the dimensions but not be controlled by them. Check out how you feel inside the mirror, if your clothing match, or whether you need to push a knot on your belt. These are all perfect measures of the greater changes in body composition.

Be mindful of other improvements, too, such as well-being, energy levels, and how clean the skin appears. At the local pharmacy, you can get tests of your general cardiovascular and metabolic well-being to see improvements in factors like blood pressure, blood sugar levels, and blood fats like cholesterol and triglycerides. Remember, weight loss aside, introducing Sirtfoods into your diet is a huge step in making your cells fitter and more disease resistant, setting you up for an exceptional healthy lifetime.

How to follow phase 1.

To make Step 1 sailing as simple as possible, we will lead you one day at a time through the full seven-day schedule, including the Sirtfood Green Juice lowdown and quick to follow tasty recipes every step of the way.

Phase 1 of the Sirtfood Diet is built on two specific stages:

Days one to three are the highest demanding, and during this time you can consume up to a limit of 1,000 calories per day, consisting of:

- Three times Sirtfood green juices
- One-time vital meal

Days four to seven will see your food consumption increase to a limit of 1,500 calories per day, consisting of the following:

- Two times Sirtfood green juices
- Two times vital meals

There are very few rules by which to obey the diet. Ultimately, for sustained progress, it's about incorporating it into the lifestyle and around daily life. But here are a few easy but major effect tips to get the best result:

1. Get a Good Juicer: Juicing is an important aspect of the Sirtfood Diet, and a juicer is one of the best health-care purchases you can make. Although the budget will be the decisive factor, some juicers are more powerful at extracting the juice from green leafy vegetables and herbs, with the Breville brand among the best juicers we've tested.

2. Preparation Is Key: One thing is evident from the abundance of reviews we've had: the most effective were those who prepared ahead of time. Get to know the ingredients and recipes, and stock up with what's needed. You'll be surprised at how simple the entire cycle is, with everything planned and ready.

3. Save Time: Prepare cleverly when you're tight on time. Meals should be rendered the previous night. Juices can be made in bulk and stored in the refrigerator for up to three days (or longer in the freezer) until their sirtuin-activating nutrient levels begin to decline. Just shield it from light, and add only when you're able to eat it in the matcha.

4. Eat Early: It's better to eat sooner in the day, and preferably, you shouldn't eat meals and salads later than 7 p.m., yet basically, the plan is designed to fit the lifestyle, so late eaters still get great benefit.

5. Space Out the Juices: They should be eaten at least one hour before or two hours after a meal to maximize the absorption of green juices and distributed throughout the day, rather than being too close together.

6. Eat to Satisfied: Sirtfoods can have drastic effects on appetite, and certain people will be satisfied before their meals are over. Listen to your body and feed until full, instead of pushing down all the calories. Tell, "Hara Hachi bu," as the long-lived Okinawans had, approximately translates to "Eat until you're 80% full."

7. Enjoy the Ride: Don't get stuck on the end goal, but keep mindful of the trip instead. This diet is about enjoying food in all its glory, for its health benefits but also for the fun and pleasure it offers. Evidence suggests that we are much more likely to succeed if we keep our eyes focused on the road rather than the ultimate goal.

What to Drink

As well as the required daily servings of green juices, other beverages can be easily drunk in Step 1. Those should be non-calorie foods, ideally straight coke, black coffee, and green tea. If your usual tastes are for black or herbal teas, do not hesitate to add these too. Apple juices and soft drinks are left behind. Instead, consider adding a few sliced strawberries to still or sparkling water to make your Sirtfood-infused health cocktail, if you want to spice things up.

Hold it for a few hours in the fridge, and you can have a surprisingly cooling alternative to soft drinks and juices. One thing you ought to be mindful of is that we don't suggest abrupt major improvements to your daily coffee use. Caffeine withdrawal symptoms may make you feel lousy for a few days; likewise, large increases may be unpleasant for those especially sensitive to caffeine effects. Since some researchers have found that adding milk will reduce the absorption of beneficial nutrients that activate sirtuin, we also recommend drinking coffee black without adding milk. The same has been found for green tea, although adding some lemon juice increases its nutrient absorption to activate sirtuin.

Remember that this is the period of hyper-success, and while you can be comforted by the fact that it is just for a week, you need to be a bit more careful. We have alcohol for this week, in the form of red wine but only as a cooking ingredient.

The Sirtfood Green Juice

The green juice is an integral component of the Sirtfood Diet's Step 1 program. All the ingredients are powerful Sirtfoods, and in every juice, you get a potent cocktail of natural compounds like apigenin, kaempferol, luteolin, quercetin, and EGCG that work together to switch on your sirtuin genes and promote fat loss. To that, we have added lemon, as it has been shown that its natural acidity prevents, stabilizes and improves the absorption of the sirtuin-activating nutrients. We added a touch of apple and ginger to taste too. But all of these are available. Indeed, many people notice that they take the apple out entirely until they become used to the flavor of the fruit.

Sirt Food Green Juice (Serves 1)

- a big handful (1 ounce or 30g) arugula
- 2 big handfuls (about 21/2 ounces or 75g) kale
- 2 to 3 big celery stalks (51/2 ounces or 150g), including

leaves
- a little handful (about 1/4 ounce or 5g) _at-leaf parsley
- 1/2 - to one -inch (1 to 2.5 cm) piece of fresh ginger
- 1/2 medium of green apple
- juice of a 1/2 lemon half level teaspoon matcha powder

*Days one to three of Phase 1: combined only to the first two juices of the day;

Days four to seven of Phase 1: combined to both juices.

Note that while we weighted all the amounts exactly as described in our pilot experiment, our experience is that a handful of measures perform exceptionally well. Besides, they are better tailoring the number of nutrients to the body type of a person. Bigger people tend to have larger paws, and therefore get a proportionally higher volume of Sirtfood nutrients to suit their body size, and vice versa for smaller people.

- Put together the greens (kale, arugula, and parsley), and apply the concentrates. When juicing leafy vegetables, you should consider juicers in their potency that can vary, so you may need to juice the rest before going on to the other ingredients. The aim is to finish up with about two ounces of fluid, or around 50 ml green juice (1/4 cup).
- Celery, ginger tea. and apple tea,
- You can still peel the lemon and put it in the juicer, but squeezing the lemon into the juice by hand is much easier for. You should have a total of around one cup (250ml) of juice by this point, maybe a little more.
- Only add matcha when the juice is rendered and ready to drink. Drop a small amount of water in a cup, then add the

matcha and whisk with a fork or a spoonful of milk vigorously.

We use matcha in the first two drinks of the day, as it contains mild levels of caffeine (the same quality as a regular cup of tea). If you are not used to it, it will make you not to sleep if you drink it in late hour.

- Add the remaining juice, once the matcha is dissolved.

Give it a last stir, then be able to drink your juice. Free to put water in it, if you like.

Phase 2: Maintenance

Congratulations on concluding Sirtfood Diet Phase 1! You will now see positive progress with a weight loss and not only look slimmer and more toned but also feel revitalized and re-energized. Yeah, now what?

Having witnessed these sometimes incredible transformations ourselves, we know how often you're going to want to see much greater outcomes, not just retain all the advantages. Sirtfoods are, after all, built to eat for life. The problem is how you adapt what you did in Step 1 into your normal dietary routine. That's exactly what prompted us to create a 14-day follow-up maintenance plan designed to help you transition from Phase 1 to your more normal dietary routine, thereby helping to maintain and extend the benefits of the Diet Sirtfood.

What to expect.

You will consolidate your weight loss results during Phase 2, and continue to lose weight steadily. Also, the one surprising point we've seen with the Sirtfood Diet is that much or all of the weight people lose is from fat, and that many even add some muscle in. We would like to warn you again not to measure your success solely based on the numbers. Look in the mirror to see how you feel leaner and more toned, see how well your suits match and soak up the compliments you'll get from everyone.

Do note that as the weight loss progresses, so do the health benefits. By following the 14-day maintenance plan, you are starting to lay the foundations for a lifelong health future.

How To Follow Phase 2

The trick to success in this process is having your diet packed full of Sirtfoods. We've put together a seven-day menu plan for you to follow to make it as easy as possible, including delicious family-friendly recipes, packed with Sirtfoods every day to the rafters.

All you need to do is replicate the Seven Day Schedule twice to complete Step 2's fourteen days. For every fourteen days, your diet must consist of:

- 1 to 2 times optional Sirtfood bite snacks
- 1-time Sirtfood green juice
- 3 times balanced Sirtfood-rich meals

Once again, there are no particular guides for when you have to take these. Be soft and fit them around your day. Two basic rules of thumb are:

- Take your green juice first thing in the morning, thirty minutes before breakfast, or mid-morning.
- Make sure you eat your evening meal by 7 p.m.

Portion Sizes

During Step 2, our attention is not on calorie counting. For the average person, this is not a practical or successful approach over the long term. Instead, we concentrate on healthy servings, very well-balanced meals, and most notably, stocking up on Sirtfoods so that you can start to benefit from their fat-burning and health-promoting effects.

We've also built the meals in the plan to make them satiate, helping you feel full for longer. That, coupled with Sirtfoods' natural appetite-regulating powers, means you're not going to spend the next 14 days feeling thirsty, but instead happily relaxed, well-fed, and highly well-nourished. Just like in Phase 1, remember to listen and be guided by your appetite. When you prepare meals according to our guidelines and find that you are easily full before you finish a meal, then stop eating perfectly!

What to drink.

Throughout Step 2, you'll have to have one green juice daily. This is to keep you top with high Sirtfoods levels. Much as in Phase 1, you can easily absorb other fluids in Phase 2. Our favorite drinks include remaining plain water, homemade flavored water, coffee, and green tea. If black or white tea is your preference, feel free to indulge. The same goes for herbal teas. The great thing is that during Step 2, you will enjoy the occasional bottle of red wine. Due to its content of sirtuin-activating polyphenols, particularly resveratrol and piceatannol, red wine is a sirtfood which makes it by far the best choice of alcoholic beverage. But, with alcohol itself causing harmful effects on our fat cells, restraint is always safest, so we suggest restricting the drink to one glass of red wine with a meal for two to three days a week during Step 2.

Returning To Three Meals

You enjoyed only one or two meals a day during Phase 1, which allowed plenty of versatility when you eat your meals. Since we are all returning to a more regular schedule and the well-tested practice of three meals a day, learning about breakfast is a perfect time.

Having a healthy breakfast sets us ready for the day, raising our levels of vitality and focus. Eating earlier keeps our blood sugar and fat levels in check, in terms of our metabolism. A variety of studies point out that breakfast is a positive idea, usually finding that people who eat breakfast are often less likely to be overweight.

The explanation for this is because our body clocks inside. Our bodies ask us to feed early in expectation of when we will be busiest and need food. Yet as many as a thirds of us will miss breakfasts on every given day. It's a typical example of our crazy everyday life and the impression that there's just not enough time to eat properly. But as you will see, nothing could be further from the truth with the nifty breakfasts we have laid out for you. If it's the Sirtfood smoothie that can be drunk on the go, the premade Sirt muesli, or the fast and simple Sirtfood scrambled eggs/tofu, having those extra few minutes in the morning will yield rewards not only for your day but also for your weight and well-being over the longer term.

With Sirtfoods working to overcharge our energy levels, there's, even more, to gain from getting a hit from them early in the morning to start your day. It is done not only by eating a Sirtfood-rich meal but also by consuming the green juice, which we suggest you have either first thing in the morning — at least thirty minutes before a meal — or mid-morning. We get a lot of stories from our personal experience about people who first drink their green juice and don't feel hungry for a few hours afterward. When this is the impact, it's having on you, waiting a couple of hours before getting breakfast is completely good. Just don't miss this one.

Alternatively, with a good breakfast, kick off your day, then wait two or three hours to have the green juice. Be flexible, and simply go with anything that works for you.

Sirtfood bites.

You should handle it when it comes to snacking or leave it. There has been too much debate about whether eating regular, smaller meals is better for weight loss, or only sticking to three healthy meals a day. The fact is, it just does not matter.

The way we've built the maintenance menu ensures you're going to eat three well-balanced Sirtfood-rich meals a day, and you might find that you don't need a snack. So maybe you've been busy with the kids in the classroom, working out or dashing about and need something to take until the next meal. And if that "little thing" would give you a whammy of Sirtfood nutrients and wonderful taste, then it's happy days. That's why we developed our "Sirtfood Bits." These fun little treats are a truly guilt-free treat made entirely from sirtfoods: almonds, walnuts, chocolate, extra virgin olive oil, and turmeric. We consider eating one, or a maximum of two, every day on the days when you need them.

'Sirtifying' Your Meals

We found that the only consistent diets are ones of inclusion, not exclusion. But real achievement goes beyond this — the diet needs to be consistent with life in modern times. If it's the ease of satisfying the demands of our hectic lives or fitting in with our position at dinner parties as to the bon vivant, the way we eat should be trouble-free. You will enjoy your svelte body and beautiful smile, rather than thinking about the demands and limitations of kooky products.

What makes Sirtfoods so awesome is that they are very available, familiar, and easy to include in your diet. Here, when you cross the distance between step 1 and daily feeding, you can lay the groundwork for a new, enhanced lifelong feeding strategy.

The key principle is what we call your meals, "Sirtifying." This is where we take popular meals, including several classic classics, and we retain all the great flavor with some smart swaps and easy Sirtfood inclusions but add a lot of goodness to that. You'll see exactly how quickly that is done during Step 2.

Examples include our tasty smoothie Sirtfood for the perfect on-the-go breakfast in a time-consuming environment and the easy turn from wheat to buckwheat to bring extra flavor and zip to the much-loved pasta comfort food. Meanwhile, iconic, beloved dishes such as chili con carne and curry don't even need much change, with Sirtfood bonanzas offering traditional recipes. And who has said that fast food means bad food? We add a pizza's authentic colorful áavors and remove the shame when you make one yourself. There's no need to say goodbye to indulgence either, as our smothered pancakes with berries and dark chocolate sauce have proved. It's not just a dessert, it's breakfast, and for you it's perfect. Easy changes: you keep eating the food that you enjoy when maintaining a good weight and well-being. And that is Sirtfoods, the dietary revolution.

To sum it up all, the Sirtfood Diet will help you:

The Sirtfood Diet is full of healthy foods, but eating patterns are not good.

Its theory and health claims are, not to mention, based on great extrapolations from preliminary scientific evidence.

While it isn't a bad to add some sirt foods to your diet and may even offer some health benefits, the diet itself looks like just another fad.

Save yourself the money and skip instead to make healthy, long-term changes to your diet.

- Lose weight, not muscle, by burning fat.
- Burn fat to fuel better health, especially from the stomach area.
- Prep the body for long-term results in weight loss.
- Sleep stronger and look better and have more time.
- Prevent strict restrictions on calories or serious hunger.
- Be free from grueling programs of fitness.
- Living a longer, healthier and sicker life

CHAPTER SIX

BUILDING A DIET THAT WORKS

We were doing something very special with the Sirtfood Diet. We took the most powerful Sirtfoods on the planet and woven them into a brand-new way of eating, the likes of which were never seen before. We selected the "best of the best" from the healthiest diets we have ever known and created a world-beating diet from them.

The good news is, you don't suddenly have to adopt an Okinawan's traditional diet or cook like an Italian mamma. That on the Sirtfood Diet is not only utterly unrealistic but unnecessary. Indeed, one thing you may be struck by from the Sirtfoods list is their familiarity. While you do not consume any of the items on the list at the moment, you are most likely eating others. Then why don't you just lose weight already?

The response is sought when we explore the various elements that the most cutting-edge nutrition research indicates are required to create a workable diet. It is about eating the right amount of Sirtfoods, range, and shape. It's about adding generous protein servings to the Sirtfood dishes and eating your meals at the best time of day. And it's about the right to consume the authentic savory foods you love in the amounts you want.

Hitting your quota.

Most people just don't consume nearly enough Sirtfoods right now to elicit a potent fat-burning and health-boosting effect.

When researchers looked at the consumption of five key nutrient-activating sirtuins (quercetin, myricetin, kaempferol, luteolin, and apigenin) in the US diet, individual daily intakes were found to be miserably 13 milligrams a day. Conversely, the average Japanese intake was five times higher. Compare this with our Sirtfood Diet trial, where everyday individuals consumed hundreds of milligrams of sirtuin-activating nutrients.

We are discussing a total diet revolution in which we increase our daily intake of sirtuin-activating nutrients by as much as heavy folding. Although that might sound overwhelming or unrealistic, it isn't necessarily. By taking all our top Sirtfoods and putting them together in a fully compatible way with your busy life, you can easily and effectively reach the intake level needed to reap all of the benefits.

The synergy Strength.

We believe it is better to consume a wide range of these wonder nutrients as whole natural foods, where they coexist alongside the hundreds of other natural bioactive plant chemicals that act synergistically to boost our health. We think working with nature is better, rather than against it. For this purpose, single-nutrient supplements do not display permanent value time and time again, but the same nutrient is given in the form of a whole diet.

Take, for example, the classic nutrient resveratrol, which activates sirtuin. It is poorly consumed in supplementary form, but its bioavailability (how much the body can use) is at least six times higher in its natural food matrix of red wine. Add to this the fact that red wine produces not only one but a whole variety of sirtuin-activating polyphenols that act together to offer health benefits, including piceatannol, quercetin, myricetin, and epicatechin. Perhaps we might turn our attention from the turmeric to curcumin.

Curcumin is well-established as the key sirtuin-activating nutrient in turmeric. Yet, research shows that whole turmeric has better PPAR-ÿ activity to fight fat loss and is more effective in inhibiting cancer and lowering blood sugar levels than isolated curcumin. It's not hard to see why isolating a single nutrient in its entire food form is nowhere near as effective as consuming it.

But what makes a dietary approach special is when we start combining multiple Sirtfoods. For example, we further enhance the bioavailability of resveratrol-containing foods by adding it to quercetin-rich Sirtfoods. Not only this, but they complement each other with their acts. Both are fat busters, but there are shades of how each of them is doing this. Resveratrol is very effective in helping destroy existing fat cells, while quercetin excels in preventing the formation of new fat cells. They target fat from both sides, resulting in a greater impact on fat loss than just eating large amounts of a single food.

And this is a trend which we see again and again. Foods rich in sirtuin activator apigenin improve quercetin absorption from food and improve its action. Quercetin, in effect, is synergistic with epigallocatechin gallate (EGCG) activity. And EGCG 's work with curcumin has been seen to be synergistic. And so it continues. Not only are individual whole foods more powerful than isolated nutrients, but we tap into a whole tapestry of health benefits that nature has weaved — so complex, so refined, it's impossible to try to trump it.

Juicing and Food: Get the Best of Both Worlds

Sirtfood Diet is composed of both juices and whole foods.

Here we are talking about juices made specifically from a juicer — blenders and smoothie makers (such as the NutriBullet) will not work. For many, this will seem counterintuitive, because the fiber is removed when something is juiced. But this is exactly what we want for leafy greens.

Food fiber includes what is called non-extractable polyphenols (or NEPPs), which are polyphenols, called sirtuin activators, which are bound to the fibrous portion of the food and only activated by our friendly gut bacteria when broken down. They don't get the NEPPs by cutting the yarn, so miss out on their beauty. Importantly, however, the NEPP content varies dramatically depending on the plant type. The NEPP content of foods such as fruits, cereals, and nuts, and these are significant.

It should be eaten whole (NEPPs provide over 50 percent of polyphenols in strawberries!). Yet, for leafy vegetables, the active ingredients in the Sirtfood juice are much lower, despite high fiber content.

When it comes to leafy greens, by juicing and eliminating the low-nutrient fiber we get full bang for our dollar, so we can use even greater amounts and obtain a super-concentrated hit of sirtuin-activating polyphenols.

There's another advantage in removing the fiber, too. Leafy greens contain a form of fiber called insoluble fiber, which has a digestive scrubbing effect. Yet when we eat so much of it, it will irritate and hurt our gut lining much as if we over-scrub stuff. That means that for many people, leafy green-packed smoothies will overload fiber, potentially aggravating or even causing IBS (irritable bowel syndrome) and hampering our nutrient absorption.

When it comes to consuming their goodness, keeping some of the Sirtfoods in juice shape can also have major advantages. E.g., a match green tea is one of the ingredients we use in the green juice. When we eat the EGCG sirtuin activator present in high amounts of green tea in the form of beverages without milk, its absorption is higher than 65 percent. We have, and it is important to remember that transitioning from smoothies to green juices caused drastic changes in their levels of other vital nutrients, such as magnesium and folic acid, when we ran blood testing on our customers.

The crux of all this is that to have the sirtuin genes going for drastic weight loss and wellbeing, and we need to develop a diet that incorporates juices and whole food for full gain.

The Power of Protein

It's plants that put the Sirt into the Sirtfood Diet, but Sirtfood meals should always be rich in protein to reap maximum benefit. It has been shown that a building block of the dietary protein called leucine has additional benefits in stimulating SIRT1 to increase fat burning and improve blood sugar control.

But leucine also has another role, and this is where it shines through its synergistic relationship with Sirtfoods. Leucine powerfully stimulates anabolism (building things) in our cells, especially in the muscle, which demands a great deal of energy and means that our energy factories (called mitochondria) have to work overtime. This creates a need for the Sirtfoods activity within our cells. As you can remember, one of the effects of Sirtfoods is to stimulate the development of more mitochondria, to increase their performance, and to make them burn fat as fuel. Our bodies, therefore, need these to meet this extra demand for energy. The upshot is that we see a synergistic effect by combining Sirtfoods with dietary protein that boosts sirtuin activation and ultimately gets you to burn fat to fuel muscle growth and healthier health.

That is why the meals in the book are meant to give you a generous meat holds.

Oily fish is an extraordinarily good protein alternative to supplement Sirtfoods' action since they are high in omega-3 fatty acids alongside their protein content. There is no question that you may have read a lot about the health effects of fatty fish and especially omega 3 fish oils. And now recent research suggests that the benefits of omega-3 fats may come from improving the workings of our sirtuin genes.

In recent years, concerns have been raised about the negative effects of protein-rich diets on health, and without Sirtfoods to counterbalance the protein, we can start to understand why. Leucine may be a knife with two-edges. We need Sirtfoods, as we have shown, to help our cells fulfill the metabolic demand that leucine imposes upon them. Without them, though, our mitochondria can become unstable, and elevated levels of leucine will potentially promote obesity and insulin resistance, rather than improve wellbeing. Sirtfoods help not only keep the symptoms of leucine in check but also work effectively in our favor.

Think of leucine as putting the foot on the weight loss and wellness engine, with Sirtfoods, the unit that ensures that the cell meets the increased demand. The engine blows, without the Sirtfoods.

Returning to questions about the safety consequences of protein-rich diets, the missing piece of the puzzle is Sirtfoods. Usually, the US diet is protein-rich but lacks Sirtfoods to counterbalance it. That makes it important for Sirtfoods to become an integral part of how Americans eat.

Eat Early

Our philosophy is the earlier, the better when it comes to eating, ideally finishing eating for the day by 7 p.m. This is on two floors. Firstly, to reap the Sirtfoods natural satiating effect.

Eating a meal that will make you feel full, happy, and energized as you go through your day is even more effective than spending the whole day feeling hungry enough to feed and stay full while you sleep through the night.

Yet there's a second good explanation to maintain eating habits in line with your inner body clock. We also have an internal body clock, called our circadian rhythm, which controls all of our normal body functions according to day time.

It affects, among other things, how the body treats the food we consume. Our clocks operate in synchrony, above all observing the signals of the sun's light-dark period. We 're designed as a diurnal species to be active in the daytime rather than at night.

Our body clock then allows us to manage food more effectively throughout the day, while it's bright, so we're supposed to be busy, and less so when it's the night when we're prepared for rest and sleep instead.

The question is that all of us have "work clocks" and "social clocks," which are not aligned with the sun's slowing down. Even after dark is the last option, any of us get to sleep. To some extent, we can train our body clock to synchronize with various schedules, like "evening chorotypes" who want to be busy, feed, and sleep later in the day. Living misaligned from the light-dark external process, however, comes at a premium.

Studies found that evening chorotype individuals have increased their sensitivity to weight accumulation, muscle loss, found metabolic issues, and sometimes had bad sleep conditions. That's exactly what we see among night-shift workers, who have higher rates of obesity and metabolic disease, at least partially due to the effects of their late eating patterns.

The upshot is that you 're best off eating early in the day, preferably by 7 p.m. But what if it is not feasible? The good news is that sirtuins play a vital role in synchronizing the body clock. Work has found that the polyphenols in Sirtfoods can modulate our body clocks and change circadian rhythm positively.

That means the inclusion of Sirtfoods with your meal will minimize the detrimental effects if you simply cannot avoid eating later on. Indeed, one of the frequent feedback we receive from Sirtfood Diet followers is their level of sleep has increased, indicating potent effects on their circadian rhythm harmonization.

Go big on taste.

A major flaw with the traditional diet is that it usually makes the eating experience unpleasant. It steals the last drop of food satisfaction and leaves us feeling sad. But for us, it's important that in maintaining a healthier weight, you retain the pleasure of food.

That's why we were pleased when we learned that Sirtfoods and foods that improve their operation like protein and omega-3 food sources are prepared to fulfill our taste desire. It's the biggest win-win: The Sirtfood diet is improving our wellbeing and fantastic tastes.

Let's go back one step to see how this works. The taste buds decide how good we and the meals are, and how happy we are at enjoying it. Seven major receptors do this to the taste.

Human beings have evolved over countless generations to seek out the tastes that stimulate these receptors to achieve maximum nutrition. The more those taste receptors are activated by a dish, the more pleasure we get from a meal. And we have the best menu in the Sirtfood Diet for healthy taste buds, as it provides full relaxation to all taste receptors. To summarize these tastes and the things you'll have on the diet that fulfill them: the seven main sensations of taste are sweet (strawberries, dates); salty (celery, fish); sour (strawberries); spicy (cocoa, kale, endive, extra virgin olive oil, green tea); pungent (chilies, garlic, extra virgin olive oil); astringent (green tea, red wine); and umami (soy, rice, meat).

We have found that the greater a food's sirtuin-activating effects, the more it activates those taste centers and the more pleasure we get from the food we consume. Importantly, it also ensures our hunger is met sooner, and our urge to consume more is that accordingly. That is a primary explanation of why those eating a Sirtfood-rich diet are quicker happily fuller.

Real cocoa, for example, has a compelling, pleasing bitter flavor, but extract the sirtuin-activating flavanols using vigorous industrial food processing methods. We are left with mass-produced, bland, and characterless cocoa that is used to manufacture heavily sweetened chocolate pastries. The health benefits have faded by this point.

The same is true of olive oil. Consumed in its minimally refined form — extra virgin — has a strong and distinct taste that can be felt at the back of the throat with a hard blow. Yet refined and processed olive oil loses all character, is mild and bland, and does not carry a kick like this. Similarly, hot chilies boast much more sirtuin-activating credentials than the milder varieties, and wild strawberries are much more tasteful than farmed ones because of richer sirtuin-activating nutritional content.

Not only that, but we can also trigger multiple taste receptors as well as individual Sirtfoods: green tea is both bitter and astringent, and strawberries have a combination of sweet and sour flavors. Initially, some palates won't get used to some of these flavors — so much of our modern food is devoid of both nutrients and true taste — but you'll be amazed at how quickly you gain a love for them. After all, humans have evolved to look for a diet rich in Sirtfoods, alongside healthy protein and omega-3 fatty acids, to satisfy our appetite's basic desires and, in turn, our health. This evolutionary process has been going on for millennia without us knowing the reasons, yet it has ensured that we get the maximum benefit from eating these foods.

Embrace Eating

Let's give an experiment a shot. We just want you to do us one very easy thing: don't worry about a white bear.

What do you think? For example, a white rabbit. Why? For what? Since we told you they didn't. Don't tell us you're already there!

This was the trailblazing experiment performed in 1987 by psychology professor Daniel Wegner, which revealed that coerced repression of thoughts leads to a paradoxical and detrimental increase of how much we think about what we are attempting to suppress. And rather than blocking it from our minds, the action creates compassion for the silenced feeling.

And as you've already noticed, this trend doesn't even refer to white bears. The very same thing happens when we are making heroes and limiting weight loss products. Studies suggest that in general, we think more frequently of them, raising the temptation. It's chewing again before we eat it! And now we are much more likely to binge with the diet disrupted and the heightened anxiety of the "forbidden" foods we have experienced.

Now the physicists have explained what's going on here. We also need to be fully autonomous. When we feel restricted, like going on a strict diet, this creates a negative atmosphere, making us feel uncomfortable. We get wrapped up in this misery, and we fight to get out. We protest by doing what we've been told we shouldn't be doing, and doing so much more than we should have at first. It happens to us all, even to the most self-controlled ones.

It's not a case of when nor if. Scientists now agree that this is a key explanation that we can sustain diets and even see early effects but struggle to achieve long-term progress. And does this mean that there is no point in ever trying to change our eating habits? Are we all destined to fail? No, it means that we need to make our own optimistic, ideal decision while making a transition to success. We now realize that it is not through dietary exclusion but through dietary inclusion that we can do it. Instead of concentrating your attention on the negatives of what you shouldn't consume, then concentrate on the good qualities of what you should consume. You escape the social reaction by doing so. And the Sirtfood Diet's elegance is this. It's just what you put in your diet and not what you're throwing out. It's about consistency and not the quantity of your food.

And it's about you having to do so because you feel good eating great-tasting foods with the additional awareness that every bite offers a wealth of advantages.

Many diets represent a means to an end. They're about hanging in there, striving to keep track of the "thin dream." But it never happens until the diet stalls, so it's never maintained, even if accomplished. There's a particular Sirtfood Diet. It's just for flying. Step 1, which reduces calories, is kept purposely short and quick to ensure positive effects are done before any adverse reaction happens. The priority then is solely on Sirtfoods. And the desire to eat Sirtfoods isn't just motivated by an end product of weight loss. But it is just as much if not more about appreciating and loving real food for a safe, comfortable lifestyle.

What's more, if you take advantage of Sirtfoods' specific advantages, from fulfilling your hunger to improving your quality of life, you can change your preferences and tastes. With the Sirtfood Diet, foods that would have traditionally set off the chain of adverse responses if you were advised that you couldn't eat them would lose their appeal and diminish their hold. They are a tiny part of the diet, and everything has been done without

Just one white bear sighting.

Chapter seven

Sirtfood with other food

As we traveled deeper and deeper into Sirtfoods' wonderful universe, we started to understand how big their application could be. We are well aware that no two people eat the same. Many health-conscious individuals are firmly dedicated to any form of eating, with the likes of paleo, low-carbon, intermittent fasting, and gluten-free diets becoming especially common. Although for others they aren't effective, some swear by them.

But how will these blend into Sirtfoods?

A lightbulb moment struck with the understanding that if Sirtfoods were introduced into them, any one of those common diets would be greatly enhanced. The advantages people obtained from the health or weight loss can be increased in adequate amounts by adding Sirtfoods. Sirtfoods are similar in respect: if there is a way to eat that does well for you, adding Sirtfoods into it will make the results much better.

We 're both busy physicians, so our passion for Sirtfoods has evolved. We've steadily incorporated Sirtfoods into the diets of the clients we deal with, irrespective of their favorite eating process. Our inference is clear: Sirtfoods are consistent with all other nutritional strategies, but they are also effectively enhancing. Indeed in any common diet, they should be important ingredients.

Overlook them, and you lose a trick.

LOW-CARB DIET

Low-carb diets have been a significant trend on the weight-loss map ever since Atkins, the founder of low-carb diets, rose to meteoric prominence. Subsequent reincarnations have tended to power the low-carb trend, such as the Dukan diet. Between them, they have notched up to tens of millions in diet-book sales. While these low-carb diets can be severe, especially in their early phases of "attack," their strong feelings reflect a broader change in opinion towards an anti-sugar and even anti-carbon stance. Citizens are gradually fleeing the sinking ship of the low-fat ideology, and the changing loyalties towards the "carbs are the enemy" camp.

One of the Sirtfood Diet 's uniqueness is that it doesn't include this territorial dispute. It's an inclusive diet, which ensures you don't have to pick sides to remove a whole range of foods from your lifestyle to reach the body you desire. Nonetheless, we know that many people choose a lower-carb eating style, so where does Sirtfoods come in?

If you are encouraged to be low-carb, we advise you not to scrimp on Sirtfoods, but to accept them. Some of the main pitfalls we find in people slipping into when eating low-carb diets in our professional practice is the shortage of plant-based ingredients that they provide. Meals are largely focused around meat (most sometimes refined beef), fish, milk, cheese, and other dairy products, and vegetable-based diets are confined to the bottom of the pecking order. Yet if it's low carb, we 're told it's all fine, or so.

Sadly, faced with nearly everything we know about nutrition and health, the belief that plant-based foods are not vital in our diets flies. A diet stripped from the overwhelming amount of healthy compounds present in plant foods can do nothing to avert an explosion of infectious disorders such as diabetes, heart disease, and cancer. And the surplus of Sirtfoods can easily be blended into a carb-restricted way of eating. Only look at the top twenty Sirtfoods list, and you'll figure that a huge majority of them are relatively weak in carbohydrates. We are talking of an abundance of leafy and low-carb vegetables (arugula, celery, endive, cabbage, onions), culinary herbs (garlic, parsley), spices (chili, turmeric), capers, walnuts, chocolate, and extra virgin olive oil, not to mention the drinks (coffee and green tea). As for fruit, too much the focus of targeting low-carb diets, even the strawberries weigh in a generous 31/2-ounce (100 g) portion with a pure teaspoon of carbohydrates.

The bottom line for us is this: a low-carb diet would not be a low-Sirtfood diet. Incorporating Sirtfoods not only improves a low-carb diet's weight-loss advantages but also significantly raises its health potential.

INTERMITTENT FASTING/THE 5:2 DIET

Over the past few years, intermittent fasting, also known as IF, has become a major culinary trend, epitomized by the 5:2 diet's runaway popularity. That usually includes restricting calorie consumption on two days a week to between 500 and 600 calories a day and consuming whatever you want on the other five days.

While solid work on the effects of intermittent fasting is still very limited, it does seem to be helpful for weight loss and boost some of the disease risk factors. But as we have shown, it is not appropriate for large portions of the population, it induces unnecessary loss of muscle, and it is only successful if you can stick to it. And that's always the elephant in the house when it comes to extended fasting and why we don't enjoy it so much. In our clinical context, for some considerable amount of time, most individuals refuse to adhere to intermittent fasting regimens. Hunger is an uncomfortable sensation that is gnawing away at you, and naturally, people don't like getting hungry.

Although intermittent fasting hasn't turned out to be a panacea, it's popular for a cause, and fans would swear by its advantages. Of course, we appreciate this. But why not make a major improvement to your fast by "Sirtifying" it?

With the addition of Sirtfoods, you will get all the advantages they offer, from helping to satiate hunger and conserve muscle, to reduce the negative effects of fasting. But their presence has yet another major bonus. You'll note that fasting 's benefits are induced by triggering our sirtuin genes, which is also exactly how Sirtfoods function. That means you can boost your calorie intake to a far more achievable amount while still reaping all the same benefits with Sirtfoods now present to share the fasting "burden."

That is exactly what we find in our clinical experience. Followers have been able to raise their energy consumption from an extreme 500 to 600 calories on quick days to a far more achievable 800 to 1,000 calories with only the addition of Sirtfood-rich green juices (the same recipe included in this book) into a regular IF diet.

And if your penchant is for extended fasting, by not accepting Sirtfoods, you 're losing a trick and making short days unduly grueling. There's also a whole new perspective from which intermittent fasting diets will benefit from accepting Sirtfoods.

There is very little if any, emphasis on the consistency of the food for IF diets; it's just about the calorie loss on the fast days. The proponents are vociferous in supporting the notion that on non-fast days you should eat whatever you want. It doesn't even seem to care if what you eat is good, mediocre, or awful. Yet, as we know, to keep anything running in tip-top condition, the body requires a constant supply of vital nutrients. Can we hope to get away with depriving the body of vital calories by eating whatever nutrient-stripped, refined foods we choose, particularly though we fast for two days and stay away from chronic diseases such as Alzheimer's or heart disease?

What if, on the other hand, nutrient-dense Sirtfoods were also used on your non-fasting days? You will no doubt be eating fat and just two days a week enhancing your health — it will be seven today. To us, this development of the sporadic approach to fasting is a no-brainer. It's the equivalent to replacing a full-color HD black-and-white Set.

PALEO DIET

In a nutshell, the paleo diet advocates the belief that before the introduction of western agriculture and more recently industrial food production, we would consume the diets that our ancestors were meant to consume. Essentially we 're talking of a diet-style hunter-gatherer or caveman consisting of meats, seafood, shellfish, vegetables, fruits, and nuts, while banished to the forest are dairy foods, cereal grains, starch, and other refined food.

They raise this question for paleo dieters: what could be more paleo than consuming the plant foods from which we have coevolved that turn on our ancient sirtuin genes? You must note that both plants and animals have evolved ways to deal with frequent environmental pressures such as drought, exposure to the sun, lack of nutrients, and aggressor attacks. Plants have evolved particularly sophisticated stress-response mechanisms because of their sedentary nature (they can't run away!), creating a complex assortment of polyphenols that allow them to cope with their environment. These polyphenols have been eaten by humans for decades, piggybacking on these sophisticated plant-produced stress-response signals and reaping huge benefits as they turn to our sirtuin genes.

How might we more paleo than drinking the plant-activating sirtuin compounds on which our hunter-gatherer forebears thrived? The missing piece of paleo theory is sirtfoods.

GLUTEN-FREE DIET

For those wanting to stop gluten, the advantage of the Sirtfood Diet is that the top twenty Sirtfoods are all naturally gluten-free. Gluten is a protein that is present in maize, rye, and barley.

Many individuals with a gluten allergy (through cross-contamination) may also be prone to oats. The autoimmune celiac disorder, affecting as much as 1 in 100 people in America, is hypersensitive to gluten and cannot be ingested in some way. Yet, apart from this very severe gluten allergy, several citizens are progressively experiencing gluten-free.

Diets and sometimes they have a great outlook on them.

As people embark on gluten-free diets, which include taking out staples like bread, pasta, and the myriad of other foods made from gluten-containing grains, one of the major issues is that the diet is nutritionally deficient and no longer offers the full variety of nutrients and fibers needed to stay in good health. What's so amazing about the Sirtfood Diet is that one of our top Sirtfoods is buckwheat, a naturally gluten-free and highly nutritious pseudo-grain, which, as we've seen in the previous chapters, is flexible enough to serve as a substitute for gluten-containing grains, whether in the form of flour, pasta, flakes or noodles (check the box carefully to make sure they are 100 percent).

The better diets are, of course, the ones that are complex and interesting, not bland and monotonous. We also have shown that quinoa, another pseudo-grain, is not just gluten-free, it often has substantial quantities of sirtuin-activating nutrients, rendering it the great buckwheat replacement. Aside from its normal appearance as a plant, quinoa is widely available from natural food retailers and online niche vendors in the form of rice, chips, and pasta.

With quinoa and buckwheat taking center stage, it's happier days for those following a gluten-free diet: they provide a healthy alternative to certain grains, but they also bring some strong Sirtfood credentials the regular diet as staple products.

We cannot end the issue of gluten-free diets without a word of advice about the amount of gluten-laden processed food that is now filled in the supermarket's "free-from" shelves. They are the finely processed, dried, sugar-free, gluten-free alternatives to pies, pancakes, cookies, cereals for breakfast, etc. That has become a big industry, but please do not slip into the pit of believing that it is inherently safe only because a food is gluten-free. Most of these foods are junk nutritionally pure, just like their counterparts, which contain gluten. If you are adopting a gluten-free diet, we advise you to take your health and well-being to a whole new stage with a diet rich in naturally gluten-free syrtle foods, not gluten-free garbage.

What food you can't consume with a sirtfood diet?

Officially, there is no food you can't consume on the Sirtfood Diet, but the calorie restriction is severe especially within the first three days you're restricted to 1,000 calories.

CHAPTER EIGHT

TOP TWENTY SIRTFOODS AND BEYOND THE TOP TWENTY FOODS

Now that you know all about Sirtfoods, why they're so strong, and what it takes to build a successful diet that will produce lasting results, it's time to get started. The next chapter marks the start of day one of the Sirtfood Diet. So now is the best moment to get acquainted with each of the top twenty Sirtfoods which will quickly become the staples of your everyday diet.

Arugula

Arugula (also known as a missile, rucola, rugula, and roquette) has a vivid background of American culinary culture. A pungent green salad leaf with a distinctive peppery flavor soon ascended from humble beginnings as the base of many Mediterranean peasant dishes to becoming an emblem of food snobbery in the United States, thus contributing to the coining of the word arugulance!

Yet long before it became a salad leaf used in a battle of wealth, Arugula became valued for its healing qualities by the ancient Greeks and Romans. Commonly used as a diuretic and digestive aid, it earned its true renown from its notoriety for possessing strong aphrodisiac powers, so much so that the production of Arugula was forbidden in monasteries in the Middle Ages, and the famed Roman poet Virgil wrote that "the rocket excites the sexual appetite of drowsy men." A mixture of kaempferol and quercetin is being studied as a topical product in addition to strong sirtuin-activating effects. Together, they moisturize and promote collagen production in the skin. With those credentials, it's time to lose that elitist tag and make this the leaf of choice for salad bases, where it beautifully combines with an extra virgin olive oil dressing, combining to create a strong double act of Sirtfood.

Buckwheat

Buckwheat was one of Japan's first domesticated grains, and the legend goes that when Buddhist monks took long journeys into the mountains, they'd only bring a cooking pot and a buckwheat bag for warmth. Buckwheat is so good that this was all they wanted, and it kept them up for weeks. We 're huge fans of buckwheat too. Firstly, since it is one of a sirtuin activator's best-known origins, named rutin. But also because it has benefits as a cover crop, enhancing soil fertility and reducing weed growth, making it a perfect crop for environmentally friendly and sustainable agriculture.

The reason buckwheat is head and shoulders above other, more growing grains is possible that it's not a grain at all—it's a rhubarb-related fruit crop. Having one of the highest protein content of any grain and being a Sirtfood powerhouse, makes it an unrivaled alternative to more widely used grains. Moreover, it is as flexible as any grain, and being naturally gluten-free, it is a perfect alternative for those intolerant to gluten.

Capers

In case you 're not so familiar with capers, we 're talking about the spicy, dark green, pellet-like stuff on top of a pizza that you may never have had occasion to see. But certainly, they are one of the most undervalued and neglected foods out there.

Intriguingly, they are the caper bush's flower buds that grow abundantly in the Mediterranean before being picked and preserved by hand. Studies now show that capers possess essential antimicrobial, antidiabetic, anti-inflammatory, immunomodulatory, and antiviral properties, and have a long tradition of being used as a medicine in the Mediterranean and North Africa. It's hardly shocking when we find that they are filled with nutrients that trigger sirtuin.

We think it is about time these tiny morsels got their share of fame, too much overlooked by the other big hitters from the Mediterranean diet. Flavor-wise it's a matter of huge things coming in little bags because they're confident they 're kicking. But if you don't know how to use them, then don't feel scared. We'll have you up to speed and head down soon

Over heels for these diminutive nutrient superstars, who have a remarkably identifiable and inimitable sour/salty taste when paired with the right ingredients to finish off a meal in style.

Celery

For millennia, Celery was around and revered — with leaves found adorning the remains of the Egyptian pharaoh Tutankhamun who died around 1323 BCE. Early varieties were very bitter, and Celery was commonly considered a medicinal plant, particularly for washing and detoxification to prevent disease. This is especially interesting considering that the protection of liver, kidneys, and intestines is one of the many positive benefits

Technology is now showing itself. Throughout the seventeenth century, it was domesticated as a potato, and selective breeding reduced its strong bitter flavor throughout favor of sweeter varieties, thereby securing its position as a typical salad potato.

It is important to remember when it comes to Celery, that there are two types: blanched/yellow and Pascal / green. Blanching is a procedure developed to reduce the typical bitter taste of the Celery, which has been considered too solid. This entails shading the Celery before harvesting from sunshine, resulting in a paler color and a milder flavor. What a travesty that is, for blanching dumbs down the sirtuin-activating properties of Celery as well as dumbing down the taste. Luckily, the world is shifting and consumers are seeking true and distinct flavor, turning back to the greener variety. Green Celery is the sort that we suggest you use in both the green juices and meals, with the heart and leaves being the most nutritious pieces.

Chilies

The chili has been an important part of gastronomic history worldwide for thousands of years. At one point, it's disconcerting that we'd be so enamored by it. Its pungent fire, caused by a substance called capsaicin in chilies, is developed as a mechanism of plant defense to inflict pain and dissuade predators from feasting on it, and we appreciate that. The food and our infatuation with it are almost magical.

Incredibly one study showed that eating chilies together even increases individual cooperation. And we know from a wellness perspective that their seductive heat is perfect for triggering our sirtuins and improving our metabolism. The chili's culinary applications are also limitless, making it a simple way to offer a hefty Sirtfood boost to every meal. Although we understand that not everyone is a fan of hot or spicy food, we hope we can entice you to consider adding small quantities of chilies, particularly in light of recent studies finding that those consuming spicy foods three or more days a week have a 14 percent lower mortality risk relative to those consuming them less than once a week.

The hotter the chili, the higher the Sirtfood credentials, but be careful and stick with what suits your tastes. Serrano peppers are a perfect start-they tolerable for most people when packing oil. For more seasoned oil seekers, we suggest looking for Thai chilies for optimum sirtuin-activating benefits. This can be tough to find in retail stores but can be found regularly in Asia's niche markets. Opt for deep-colored peppers, excluding any with a wrinkled and fuzzy feel.

Cocoa.

Cocoa has amazing health benefits. It's no surprise to hear that cocoa was considered a holy food for ancient cultures like the Aztecs and Mayans, and was typically reserved for the powerful and the soldiers, consumed at feasts to win allegiance and service. Indeed, there was such high respect for the cocoa bean that it was also used as a form of currency. It was normally served as a frothy beverage back then. Yet what might be a more tasty way to get our dietary allowance of cacao than by chocolate?

Unfortunately, there's no count here for the condensed, aged, and chemically sweetened milk chocolate we usually munch. We 're talking of chocolate with 85 percent solids of cocoa to earn the Sirtfood tag. Yet even then, apart from the amount of cocoa, not all chocolate is made equal. To the acidity and give it a darker color, chocolate is also treated with an alkalizing agent (known as the

Dutch process). Sadly, this process diminishes its sirtuin-activating flavanols massively, thereby seriously compromising its health-promoting quality. Fortunately, and unlike in many other nations, food labeling laws in the United States allow alkalized cocoa to be identified and labeled "alkali grown." We advocate avoiding such items, even though they boast a higher percentage of cocoa, opting for those that have not experienced Dutch processing to enjoy the true benefits of cocoa.

Coffee

What's all that about Sirtfood Coffee? We know whatever you're thinking. We will tell you that there is no mistake. Gone are the days when a twinge of remorse had to balance our enjoyment of coffee. Evidence is unambiguous: coffee is a healthy food that is bona fide. Indeed it is a real treasure chest of fantastic nutrients that trigger sirtuin. And with more than half of Americans consuming coffee every day (to the tune of $40 billion a year!), coffee enjoys the accolade of becoming America's number one source of polyphenols. The biggest irony is that the only thing we were chastised by so many fitness "experts" for doing was, in essence, the best thing we were doing about our wellbeing each day.

This is why coffee drinkers have slightly less diabetes, and lower incidence of certain tumors and neurodegenerative disease. As for that ultimate irony, coffee protects our livers and makes them healthier instead of being a toxin! And contrary to the common misconception that coffee dehydrates the body, it is now well known not to be the case, with coffee (and tea) adding very well to daily coffee drinkers' fluid intake. While we understand that coffee isn't for everybody and certain people might be very susceptible to caffeine's effects, it's for everyone who loves a cup of joe nice days.

Extra Virgin Olive oil.

Olive oil is the most popular of Mediterranean traditional diets. The olive tree is among the world's oldest-known planted plants, also known as the "immortal tree."

And after people began pressing olives in stone mortars to harvest them, the oil has been worshipped, almost 7,000 years ago. Hippocrates cited it as a cure-all; today, a few decades later, scientific medicine confidently claims the wonderful health effects. There is now a wealth of scientific data showing that regular olive oil consumption is powerfully cardio protective. It also plays a role in reducing the risk of major modern-day diseases such as diabetes, certain cancers, and osteoporosis and being associated with increased longevity.

The trick is to buy extra virgin to reap the goodness of Sirtfood in full when it comes to olive oil. Virgin olive oil is only harvested from the fruit by mechanical means in conditions that do not contribute to the oil's oxidation, so the consistency and the polyphenol content can be assured. "Extra virgin" refers to the first pressing of the fruit ("virgin" is the second pressing); it has the greatest taste, quality, and credentials of Sirtfood, and is, therefore, the one that we strongly recommend to use.

Garlic

Garlic has been considered one of Nature's miracle foods for thousands of years, with soothing and rejuvenating properties. Egyptians feed pyramid workers with garlic to enhance their immunity, avoid various illnesses, and strengthen their performance by resisting fatigue. Garlic is a potent natural antibiotic and antifungal that is sometimes used to help cure ulcers in the stomach.

Promoting the elimination of waste materials from the body will activate the lymphatic system to "detox." Besides being researched for weight reduction, it also delivers a potent heart safety punch, reducing cholesterol by around 10 percent, lowering blood pressure by 5 to 7 percent, and lowering blood and blood sugar stickiness.

And if you are concerned about the odor of garlic being off-putting, take note. Once women were asked to determine a selection of men's body odors, it was determined that all men who ate four or more garlic cloves a day had a much more appealing and friendly scent. Researchers claim this is because it is considered to be a stronger indicator of safety. And there's always mints for fresher breath, of course!

Eating garlic has a trick to get full profit. Within garlic, the Sirtfood nutrients are complemented by another main nutrient called allicin, which gives off the distinctive scent of garlic. But after actual "injury" to the bulb, allicin only occurs in garlic. When exposed to heat (cooking) or low pH (stomach acid), its composition is halted. And when preparing garlic, chop, slice, or crumble, and then allow it to sit for about ten minutes before cooking or consuming the allicin.

Green Tea (Matcha in particular).

Many would be familiar with green tea, the toast of the Orient, and ever more common in the West. With the increasing awareness of its health benefits, green tea intake is related to less cancer, heart disease, diabetes, and osteoporosis. It is believed that green tea is so healthy for us that it is largely due to its rich content of a group of strong plant compounds called catechins, the star of the show being a special form of sirtuin-activating catechin known as epigallocatechin gallate

(EGCG).

What's the fuss about matcha, though? We prefer to think of matcha on the steroids as regular green tea. In comparison to traditional green tea, which is prepared as an infusion, it is a special powdered green tea which is prepared by dissolving directly in water.

The upshot of drinking matcha is that it contains significantly higher levels of the sirtuin-activating compound EGCG than other green tea forms. Zen priests describe matcha as the "absolute mental, and medical cure [which] has the potential to make one 's life more full" if you are looking for more endorsement.

Kale

We are at heart cynics, so we are always skeptical about what drives the latest craze for superfood advertising. Is it science, or are its interests at stake? In recent years few foods have exploded as dramatically as kale on the health scene. Described as the "lean, green brassica queen" (referring to its cruciferous vegetable family), it has become the chic vegetable for which all health-lovers and foodies are gunning. Each October, there is also a National Day of the Kale. But you don't have to wait until then to show your kale pride: there are also T-shirts, with trendy slogans like "Powered by Kale" and "Highway to Kale." That's enough for us to set the alarm bells ringing.

We've done the research, packed with doubts, and we have to confess that we assume that kale enjoys her pleasures (although we don't recommend the T-shirts!). The explanation we 're pro-kale is that it contains bumper numbers of the quercetin and kaempferol sirtuin-activating nutrients, rendering it a must-include in the

Sirtfood Diet and the source of our green Sirtfood drink. What's so refreshing about kale is that kale is available everywhere, locally grown, and very affordable, unlike the usual exotic, difficult-to-source, and exorbitantly priced so-called superfoods.

Medjool Dates.

It that comes as a shock to include Medjool dates in a list of foods that encourage weight loss and promote health—especially when we tell you that Medjool dates contain a whopping 66 percent sugar. Sugar doesn't have any sirtuin-activating effects at all; instead, it has well-established connections to obesity, heart disease, and diabetes — just the reverse of what we're looking to do. Yet refined and replenished sugar is very different from sugar brought in a nature-borne vehicle supplemented with sirtuin-activating polyphenols: the date Medjool.

Medjool dates, consumed in moderation, do not have significant blood-sugar-raising effects, incomplete comparison with regular sugar. Instead, feeding them is associated with developing less diabetes and heart disease. They have been a staple food worldwide for centuries, and there has been an explosion of scientific interest in dates in recent years, which sees them emerging as a potential medicine for some diseases. This is where the Sirtfood Diet 's beauty and strength lies: it refutes the dogma and helps you to indulge in sweet things in moderation without feeling guilty.

Parsley.

Parsley is something of a culinary conundrum. It so often occurs in recipes, but too often, it's the green token man. At best, we serve a pair of chopped sprigs and tossed as an afterthought on a plate, at worst a single sprig for decorative purposes only. This way, there on the plate, it is always languishing even after we have stopped feeding. This culinary style derives from its common use in ancient Rome as a garnish for eating after meals to restore breath, rather than being part of the meal itself. And what a shame, because parsley is a fantastic food that packs a vibrant, refreshing taste full of character.

Taste aside, what makes parsley unique is that it is an outstanding source of the sirtuin-activating compound apigenin. It is a great blessing because it is rarely present in other foods in large amounts. In our minds, apigenin binds fascinatingly to the benzodiazepine receptors, allowing us to relax and get us to sleep. Stack it all up, and it's time we embraced parsley not as omnipresent nutritional confetti, but as a product of its right to reap the wonderful health benefits.

Red Endive

Endive is a pretty new kid on the block in so far as vegetables go. Tale has it that a Belgian farmer invented endive in 1830, by mistake. The farmer stored chicory roots in his cellar, and then used them as a type of coffee substitute, only to forget them. Upon his return, he discovered that white leaves had sprouted, which he found to be tender, crunchy, and rather delicious upon degustation. Endive is now grown globally, including the USA, and earns its Sirtfood badge thanks to its outstanding sirtuin activator luteolin material. And besides the proven sirtuin-activating effects, luteolin intake has been a promising path to therapy to improve sociability in autistic children.

It has a crisp texture and a sweet flavor for those new to endive, accompanied by a gentle and pleasant bitterness. If you're ever lost on how to improve endive in your diet, you can't fail by adding her leaves to a salad where her warm, tart taste gives the right bite to an extra virgin olive oil dressing based on zesty. Red is best, just like an onion, but the yellow variety can also be considered a Sirtfood. So while the red variety may sometimes be more difficult to and, you can rest assured that yellow is a perfectly appropriate alternative.

Red Onions.

Since the time of our ancient ancestors, onions have been a culinary staple, being one of the first crops grown around 5,000 years ago. With such a long tradition of use and such strong health-giving properties, many civilizations that came before us have worshipped onions. They were held particularly by the Egyptians as objects of worship, seeing their circle-within-a-circle form as indicative of everlasting existence. And the Greeks assumed that onions made athletes better. Athletes will eat their way through large quantities of oignons before the Olympic Games, even consuming the water! It's an incredible testimony to how valuable ancient dietary wisdom can be when we consider that onions earn their top twenty Sirtfood status because they're chock-full of the sirtuin-activating compound quercetin — the very compound that the sports science world has recently started actively researching and marketing to improve sports performance. So why the red ones? Simply because they have the highest amount of quercetin, but the regular yellow ones do not fall too far behind and are therefore a nice addition.

Red wine

Any list of the top twenty Sirtfoods will not be complete without the inclusion of the original Sirtfood, red wine. The French phenomenon made headlines in the early 1990s, with it being revealed that with the French seeming to do something wrong when it came to health (smoking, lack of fitness, and rich food consumption), they had lower death rates from heart disease than countries like the United States. Physicians suggested the explanation for this was the copious amount of red wine drank. Danish researchers then conducted work in 1995 to find that low-to-moderate consumption of red wine decreased death rates, while comparable amounts of beer alcohol had little effect, and equivalent concentrations of hard liquors raised death rates. Naturally, in 2003, the rich content of a bevy of sirtuin-activating nutrients from red wine was uncovered, and the rest, as they say, became history.

Yet there is much more to the remarkable resume in red wine. Red wine appears to be able to stay free from the common cold, with average wine consumers seeing an incident loss of more than 40 percent. Studies also report implications for oral hygiene and cavity protection. With moderate intake, it has also been shown to improve social networking, and out of box thought, the after-work drink among colleagues seems to have a basis in solid science to discuss work ventures.

Moderation is, of course, important. To gain from this, only limited quantities are required, and excess alcohol easily undoes the positive. The perfect spot seems to stick up to one 5-ounce drink a day for women and up to two 5-ounce drinks a day for men according to US standards. Wines from the New York region (especially pinot noir, cabernet sauvignon, and merlot) have the highest polyphenol content of the most commonly available wines to ensure optimum sirtuin-activating bang for your dollar.

Soy.

Soy products have a long tradition as an important part of the diet of many countries in Asia-Pacific, such as China, Japan, and Korea. Researchers first turned on to soy after discovering that high soy-consuming countries had substantially lower rates of certain cancers, especially breast and prostate cancers. This is believed to be attributed to a specific category of polyphenols in soybeans known as isoflavones, which can favorably affect how estrogens function in the body, like daidzein and formononetin sirtuin-activators.

Soy oil intake has also been related to a decrease in the occurrence or severity of some diseases such as cardiovascular disease, effects of menopause, and bone loss. Highly processed, nutrient-stripped soybean forms are now a ubiquitous ingredient added to numerous processed foods.

The benefits are reaped either from natural soy products such as tofu, an excellent source of vegan protein, or in a fermented form such as tempeh, natto, or our favorite, miso, a typical Japanese paste fermented with a naturally occurring fungus that results in an extreme umami taste.

Strawberries

In recent years, the fruit has been increasingly vilified, having a poor reputation in the rising enthusiasm for sugar. Luckily for berry lovers, such a malignant image couldn't be justified any worse.

While all berries are powerhouses of nutrition, strawberries are earning their top twenty Sirtfood status due to their abundance of the fisetin sirtuin activator. And now studies support regular eating strawberries to promote healthy aging, staying off Alzheimer's, cancer, diabetes, heart disease, and osteoporosis. Its sugar content is very small, a pure 31/2 ounces tablespoon of sugar.

Intriguingly, and inherently low in sugar itself, strawberries have pronounced effects on how the body handles carbohydrates. Researchers have discovered that adding strawberries to carbohydrates decreases the need for insulin, effectively transforming the meal into a constant energy releaser. And recent work also shows that eating strawberries in diabetes treatment has close results to the opioid therapy. William Butler, the great physician of the seventeenth century, wrote in praise of the strawberry: "Doubtless God should have made a better berry, but without a doubt, God never did." We can only agree.

Turmeric.

Turmeric, a cousin of ginger, is the latest kid in food trends on the block, and Google calls it the ingredient of the 2015 breakout star. While we are just turning to it nowhere in the West, it has been valued for thousands of years in Asia, for both culinary and medical reasons. Incredibly, India is generating almost the entire world's turmeric stock, eating 80 percent of it. In Asia, turmeric is used to treat skin disorders such as acne, psoriasis, dermatitis, and rash, along with the advantages of the "golden spice" Before Indian weddings, there is a ritual where the turmeric paste is added as a skincare treatment to the bride and groom but also to symbolize the warding off darkness.

One factor that prevents turmeric 's efficacy is that the main sirtuin-activating compound, curcumin, is poorly absorbed by the body when we consume it. Analysis, though, shows that we can solve this by boiling it in oil, adding fat, and adding black pepper, both of which improve its absorption drastically. It suits well with conventional Indian food, wherein curries and other spicy dishes it is usually mixed with ghee and black pepper, which once again proves that research just catches up with the age-old knowledge of conventional eating practices.

Walnuts.

Dating back to 7000 BCE, walnuts are the oldest known human-made tree product, originating in ancient Persia, where they were the property of royalty. Fast forward to the modern-day, and walnuts are a success story in the US. California is leading the way, with California's Central Valley renowned for being the prime walnut-growing region. California walnuts provide the United States with 99 percent of commercial supply and staggering three-quarters worldwide walnut trade.

Walnuts lead the way as the number one nut for health, according to the NuVal system, which ranks foods according to how nutritious they are and has been endorsed by the American College of Preventive Medicine. Yet what truly makes walnuts stand out for us is how they fly in the face of traditional thinking: they are rich in fat and calories, but well-established for weight loss and the chance of metabolic disorders like cardiovascular disease and diabetes is reduced. This is the force of triggering the sirtuin.

The recent literature revealing walnuts to be an effective anti-aging food is less well known but equally fascinating. Evidence also points to their advantages as a brain food with the ability to slow down brain aging, reduce the risk of degenerative brain diseases, and reduce physical activity deterioration with age.

Beyond The Top Twenty Sirtfoods

We've seen why Sirtfoods are so beneficial: certain plants have sophisticated stress-response mechanisms that generate compounds that cause sirtuins — the same fasting and exercise-activated fat-burning and longevity mechanism in the body. The greater the number of compounds produced by plants in response to stress, the greater the benefit we derive from their feeding. Our list of the top twenty Sirtfoods is made up of the foods that stand out because they are specially packed full of these substances, and therefore the foods that have the most exceptional potential to influence body structure and health.

But foods' sirtuin-activating results aren't a concept of everything or nothing. There are also other plants out there that contain modest amounts of sirtuin-activating nutrients. By consuming these liberally, we allow you further to increase the range and diversity of your diet. The Sirtfood Diet is all about inclusion, and the greater the range of sirtuin-activating foods that can be integrated into the diet.

This is especially so if that means you can harvest from your meals even more of your favorite foods to increase the fun and enjoyment.

Let's use the workout analogy. The top twenty Sirtfoods are the (much more pleasurable) version to working it out at the gym, with Phase 1 being the "boot camp." In comparison, eating certain other foods containing more mild amounts to sirtuin-activating nutrients is like reaping the benefits of going out for a nice stroll. Contrast it to the standard diet that has a nutritious benefit equal to sitting all day on the sofa watching Television. Yeah, sweating it out in the gym is good, but if that is everything you do, you will quickly get fed up with it. That walk should also be welcomed, particularly if you don't just want to lay on the couch.

E.g., in our top twenty Sirtfoods, we have included strawberries since they are the most prominent source of the sirtuin activator fisetin. And if we look more closely at berries as a food category, we find that they have metabolic health advantages as well as balanced aging. Reviewing their nutritional content, we find that other berries such as blackberries, black currants, blueberries, and raspberries do have significant amounts of nutrients that cause sirtuins.

The same is true to nuts. Notwithstanding their calorific material, nuts are so effective that they positively encourage weight loss and help move inches from the hips. That is in addition to reducing chronic disease risk. Although walnuts are our champion nut, nutrients that activate sirtuin can also be found in chestnuts, pecans, pistachios, and even peanuts.

Then, we turn our attention to food. In recent years there has been, in some areas, an increasing aversion to grains. Studies, however, link whole-grain intake with reduced inflammation, diabetes, heart disease, and cancer. While they do not equal the pseudo-grain buckwheat Sirtfood qualifications, we can see substantial sirtuin-activating nutrients in other whole grains. And needless to say, their sirtuin-activating nutrient content is decimated as whole grains are converted into refined "pure" forms. Such modified forms are quite a dangerous lot and are interested in some state-of-the-art safety issues. We're not suggesting you should never eat them, but instead, you're going to be way better off sticking to the whole-grain variety wherever possible. Quinoa is a decent

Sirtfood choice for those wishing to remain gluten-free. And look no further than popcorn for a perfect, whole grain Sirtfood snack that everybody enjoys.

With the likes of goji berries and chia seeds possessing Sirtfood powers, also notorious "superfoods" get on the record. That is most definitely the unwitting explanation for the health advantages they have experienced. While it does mean that they are good for us to eat, we also know that there are cheaper, more accessible, and better options out there, so don't feel compelled to jump on that particular bandwagon! We see the same trend across a lot of food classes.

Unsurprisingly, the foods that science has developed are generally healthy for us, and we should be consuming more of them.

Below we listed another forty foods that we discovered have Sirtfood properties too. They strongly urge you to add these foods to sustain and promote your weight reduction and health while you further broaden your diet collection.

Vegetables

- broccoli
- bok choy/pak choi
- asparagus
- artichokes
- yellow endive
- watercress
- white onions
- green beans
- shallots
- frisée

Fruits

- red grapes
- raspberries
- goji berries
- cranberries
- black plums
- black currants
- kumquats
- blackberries
- apples

Nuts and seeds

- sunflower seeds
- pistachio nuts
- pecan nuts
- peanuts
- chia seeds
- chestnuts

Grains and pseudo-grains

- whole-wheat flour
- quinoa
- popcorn

Beans

- white beans (e.g., cannellini or navy)
- fava beans

Herbs and spices

- ginger
- dried sage
- dried oregano
- dill (fresh and dried)
- cinnamon
- chives
- peppermint (fresh and dried)
- thyme (fresh and dried)

Beverages

- white tea
- black tea

Protein Power

A high protein diet is one of the most common diets in the last few years. Higher protein intake while dieting has been shown to encourage satiety, sustain metabolism, and reduce muscle mass loss. Yet it's when they pair Sirtfoods with protein that things get taken to a whole new level.

Protein is, as you can remember, a necessary addition in a diet focused on Sirtfood to reap full benefits. Protein consists of amino acids, and it is a particular amino acid, leucine, which effectively complements Sirtfoods' behavior, reinforcing their effects. This is achieved largely by modifying our cellular environment, so that our diet's sirtuin-activating nutrients function even more efficiently. This means we get the best outcome from a Sirtfood-based meal which is paired with protein high in leucine. Leucine's main dietary options include red meat, poultry, fish, shrimp, milk, and dairy products.

Animal based protein

Animal products have been implicated in recent years as a leading cause of many Western diseases, especially cancer. If that is the case, eating them with Sirtfoods may not seem like such a good idea. To bring that to rest, here's our lowdown.

One major worry about milk is that it is not only a basic food but also a highly sophisticated signaling mechanism to cause rapid offspring body production. While this has a cherished meaning in early life, it may not be so common in adult life.

Persistent and hyper activation of the main growth signal now correlated with aging and the progression of age-related conditions such as obesity, type 2 diabetes, cancer, and neurodegenerative diseases.

Given the intricacies of this signaling mechanism being a fairly recent field of science and, therefore, still very much an uncertain and theoretical possibility, this does explain why people would shy away from dairy products. However, evidence points to one thing: if we add Sirtfoods to a dairy diet, they inhibit the unwanted effects of mTOR on our cells, revoke this risk and make Sirtfoods a must-include

A vegetarian diet.

Overall there are mixed opinions of the association between dairy and cancer. When we stack up all the study, mild dairy intake is perfectly fine in the sense of a Sirtfood-rich diet and can deliver many useful nutrients to complement Sirtfoods.

Poultry is safe when it comes to meat and cancer risk, but red and fried meats are even more suspect. While evidence involving them in breast and prostate cancer on the ground is quite thin, there is a legitimate concern that the consumption of red and processed meat plays a role in intestinal cancer.

The biggest culprit appears to be fried beef, such as ham, hot dogs, and pepperoni. Although there is no reason to take it off the table, it can be used in just limited doses, rather than being a staple.

The positive news for red meat is that evidence reveals that cooking it with Sirtfoods rescues the chance of cancer, whether it's making a marinade with herbs, spices, and extra virgin olive oil; cooking the beef with onions, or just adding a nice cup of green tea to the meal or indulging in dark chocolate after dinner.

These all pack a punch from Sirtfood, which helps to neutralize the adverse effects of red meat. Although we're all out to get the steak and eat it, don't go overboard. Red meat consumption is best kept below around 1 pound (500 g) a week (cooked weight), approximately equal to 1.5 pounds (700 to 750 g) raw.

The link between egg intake and cancer risk has not been investigated as extensively as meat and dairy products have, but there is little reason for concern. What eggs have been involved in inducing is heart disease, instead. This is because they constitute a significant dietary cholesterol source. Thus we are told to limit the use of eggs. It is interesting to note that other countries, including Nepal, Thailand, and South Africa, recommend egg consumption for their nutritional benefits as often as they do every day. Who is right, then? The evidence to siding with the latter is convincing. There is no associated routine egg intake with any elevated risk of coronary heart disease or stroke. While particular genetic disorders require a decreased intake of dietary cholesterol, this limitation is not important for the general public.

The Power Of Three

The second major nutrient group that powerfully complements Sirtfoods is the omega-3 long-chain fatty acids EPA and DHA. For years omega-3s have been the cherished favorite of the nutritional health world. What we didn't know previously, which we do now, is that they also enhance the activity of a subset of sirtuin genes in the body that is directly linked to longevity. This makes them the perfect pairing with Sirtfoods.

Omega-3s have potent effects in reducing inflammation and reducing the level of fats in the blood. To that, we can add additional heart-healthy effects: they make the blood less likely to clot, stabilize the electrical rhythm of the heart, and bring down blood pressure.

Even the pharmaceutical industry is now turning to them as an aid in the battle against heart disease. And the litany of benefits doesn't end there. Omega-3s also affect the way we think, having been shown to improve mood as well as helping to stave off dementia.

When we talk about omega-3s, we're essentially talking about eating fish, specifically the oily varieties, because no other dietary source comes close to providing the significant levels of EPA and DHA we need. And all we need to see the benefits is two servings of fish a week, with an emphasis on oily fish.

Unfortunately, the United States is not a nation of big fish eaters, and fewer than one in five Americans achieve this. As a result, our intake of the precious EPA and DHA comes up woefully short.

Plant foods such as nuts, seeds, and green leafy vegetables also contain omega-3 but in a form called alpha-linolenic acid, which needs to be converted to EPA or DHA in the body. This conversion process is poor, which means that alpha-linolenic acid provides a negligible amount of our omega-3 needs. Even with the wonderful benefits from Sirtfoods, we should not overlook the added value that consuming sufficient levels of omega-3 fats brings. The best omega-3 fish sources are herring, sardines, salmon, trout, and mackerel, in that order. While fresh tuna is naturally high, the majority of the omega-3 is lost in the tinned version. And for vegetarians and vegans, while plant sources should still be incorporated into the diet, a supplement of DHA-enriched microalgae (up to 300 milligrams a day) is also encouraged.

CHAPTER NINE

❦

SIRTFOOD RECIPES

If you're talking of trying the Sirtfood Diet, we're here with some delicious Sirtfood Diet recipes to give you a helping hand. A seven-day routine to shed an average of 7 lb is also included in the book, but if you want a more flexible approach, adding Sirtfood ingredients to your diet will also help.

The Sirtfood Juice

A fast way to get started should be with the Sirtfood Juice – so we've put that in the recipe as a bonus to get you off. The book proposes that you drink three juices and add one meal for the first three days, then two juices and two meals for the next 4.Sirtfood Green Juice (serves1)

Ingredients:

- a very small handful (5g) flat-leaf parsley
- 2-3 big stalks (150g) green celery with its leaves
- large handfuls (75g) kale
- a very small handful (5g) lovage leaves (optional)
- a large handful (30g) rocket
- 1/2 level tsp matcha green tea
- juice of a 1/2 lemon
- 1/2 medium green apple

Instructions:

1. Blend the greens (kale, rocket, parsley, and lovage, if used), then sauté them. We think juicers may always vary in their performance when juicing leafy vegetables, and before going on to the other ingredients, you will have to re-juice the remaining. The target is to finish off the greens with about 50ml of water.

2. Now celery and apple juice both of them. You can even peel the lemon and bring it into the juicer, but we find it much easier to squeeze the lemon into the juice. At this stage, you will have a sum of about 250ml of juice, maybe a little more. after you make the juice available to drink you can now add the green tea matcha.

3. put small juice into a cup, then put the matcha, and stir it vigorously with a spoon or a fork. In the first two drinks of the day, we only use matcha, as it contains small caffeine (the same quality as a regular teacup). If you drink it late, it will keep you awake for people that are not used to it. If the matcha has been diluted, add the juice that is remaining.

4. Give it a last stir, and the juice is set for consumption. Free to combine with water, if you like.

Aromatic chicken breast with kale and red onions and a tomato and chili salsa (serves 1)
Ingredients:

- 1 tbsp extra virgin olive oil
- 50g kale, chopped
- 20g red onion, sliced
- 120g skinless, boneless chicken breast

- 2 tsp ground turmeric
- juice of ¼ lemon
- 1 tsp chopped fresh ginger
- Juice of ¼ lemon
- For the salsa
- 1 tbsp capers, finely chopped
- 1 bird's eye chilli, finely chopped
- 130g tomato (about 1)
- 5g parsley, finely chopped
- 50g buckwheat

Instructions:

1. Remove the eye from the tomato and slice it very finely to produce the salsa, taking care to preserve as much of the liquid as possible. Mix with the chillies, capers, lemon juice, and parsley. You could mix everything using a blender, but it might be a little different at the end.

2. Heat the oven about 220oC / gas 7. In one tablespoon of the turmeric, the lemon juice, and a little butter, marinate the chicken breast. Abandon for five to ten minutes. Heat an oven frying pan until it is hot, then add the marinated chicken and cook on each side for about a minute or so until light yellow, then put it back to the oven for eight to ten minutes or until it is cooked very well (place on a baking tray if your pan is not ovenproof). Remove it from the oven, cover it with foil, and allow to chill before serving for about five minutes.

3. In the meanwhile cook the kale for five minutes in a steamer. Fry the red onions and ginger using a small oil, until it is very smooth but colorless, then put the fried kale and fry for

another minute. Cook the buckwheat with the remaining turmeric tablespoon, as per the package instructions. Serve with chicken and onions, complete with salsa.

Sirtfood bites (makes 15-20 bites)
Ingredients:

- the scraped seeds of 1 vanilla pod or 1 tsp vanilla extract
- 30g dark chocolate (85 percent cocoa solids), broken into pieces; or cocoa nibs
- 1–2 tbsp water
- 1 tbsp extra virgin olive oil
- 1 tbsp ground turmeric
- 1 tbsp cocoa powder
- 120g walnuts
- 250g Medjool dates pitted

Instructions:

1. Place the walnuts and chocolate in a food processor and process them until the powder is perfect.

2. Add all other ingredients except water and blend until the mixture forms a circle. Depending on the consistency of the paste, you may or may not have to apply the water-you don't want it to be so wet.

3. Shape the mixture into bite-sized balls with your palms, refrigerate for at least 1 hour in an airtight jar before eating them. In some more cocoa or desiccated coconut, you could roll any of the balls to achieve a different texture if you prefer. They can be kept in a your fridge for up to one week.

Asian king prawn stir-fry with buckwheat noodles (serves 1)
Ingredients:

- 150g shelled raw king prawns, deveined
- 2 tsp extra virgin olive oil
- 2 tsp tamari (you can use soy sauce if you are not avoiding gluten)
- 75g soba (buckwheat noodles)
- 1 tsp finely chopped fresh ginger
- 1 bird's eye chilli, finely chopped
- 1 garlic clove, finely chopped
- 40g celery, trimmed and sliced
- 20g red onions, sliced
- 50g kale, roughly chopped
- 75g green beans, chopped
- 5g lovage or celery leaves
- 100ml chicken stock

Instructions:

1. Heat a frying pan over high fire, then cook the prawns for two to three minutes in one teaspoon tamari and one teaspoon oil. Place the prawns on a tray. Wipe the pan out with paper from the oven, because you will be using it again.

2. Cook the noodles for about eight to ten minutes in boiling water, or as indicated on the package. Drain and pack it aside.

3. Use the remaining oil, fry the garlic, fry the garlic, red onion, beans, celery, and kale for about two or three minutes on a high heat medium. Put the stock and continue to cook until the vegetables are cooked but crunchy, then simmer for one to two minutes.

4. Put the noodles, prawn and lovage/celery leaves to the saucepan, boil everything, you may now heat and eat it when it's ready.

ASIAN SHRIMP STIR-FRY WITH BUCKWHEAT NOODLES SERVES 1

- 1/3 pound (150g) shelled raw jumbo shrimp, deveined
- 2 teaspoons extra virgin olive oil
- 2 teaspoons tamari (or soy sauce, if you are not avoiding gluten)
- 2 garlic cloves, finely chopped
- 3 ounces (75g) soba (buckwheat noodles)
- 1 teaspoon finely chopped fresh ginger
- 1 Thai chili, finely chopped
- 1/2 cup (75g) green beans, chopped
- 1/2 cup (45g) celery including leaves, trimmed and sliced, with leaves

Set aside

- 1/8 cup (20g) red onions, sliced
- 1/2 cup (100ml) chicken stock
- 3/4 cup (50g) kale, roughly chopped

Instruction

1. Heat a frying pan over high pressure, then cook the shrimp for two to three minutes in one teaspoon tamari and one teaspoon oil. Put the shrimp into a tray. Wipe the pan clean with a towel of ink, because you will be using it soon.

2. Cook the noodles for five to eight minutes in boiling water, or as indicated on the box. Drain and pack it aside.

3. Meanwhile, in the remaining tamari and oil over medium-high heat, fry the garlic, chili, ginger, red onion, celery (but not the leaves), green beans, and kale for two to three min.

4. Add the stock and bring to a boil, then steam for a minute or two until cooked but crunchy.

5. Attach the shrimp, pasta, and leaves of celery to the pan, bring back to a boil, then remove fire and serve it.

MISO AND SESAME GLAZED TOFU WITH GINGER AND CHILI
STIR-FRIED GREENS
SERVES 1

- 1 x 5-ounce (150g) block of firm tofu
- 1/4 cup (40g) red onion, sliced
- 1 tablespoon mirin
- 1 stalk (40g) celery, trimmed (about 1/3 cup when sliced)
- 31/2 teaspoons (20g) miso paste
- 1 Thai chili
- 1 small (120g) zucchini (about 1 cup when sliced)
- 1 teaspoon finely chopped fresh ginger
- 2 garlic cloves
- 3/4 cup (50g) kale, chopped
- 2 teaspoons sesame seeds
- 1 teaspoon ground turmeric
- 1/4 cup (35g) buckwheat
- 1 teaspoon tamari (or soy sauce, if you are not avoiding gluten)
- 2 teaspoons extra virgin olive oil

Instruction

1. Heat the oven about 400oF (200oC). Line a thin, parchment-paper roasting pan.

2. Mix both the mirin and the miso. Cut the tofu in a lengthwise pattern, then diagonally split each slice into triangles in half. Cover the tofu with the miso mixture, and allow to marinate while cooking the other ingredients.

3. Slice the red onion, celery, and the courgettes into angle. Thinly chop the chili, garlic, and ginger, then set aside.

4. Boil The Kale in a steamer for about five minutes, bring the kale out and throw away the water.

5. Place the tofu in the roasting saucepan, scatter the tofu with the sesame seeds, and roast in the oven for fifteen to twenty minutes until it is well caramelized.

6. Wash the buckwheat in a sieve, then put it along with the turmeric in a saucepan of boiling water. Cook as indicated by the package, then drain.

7. Heat the oil in a frying pan; add the celery, onion, zucchini, chili, garlic, and ginger and fry over high heat for one to two minutes, then reduce to medium heat for three to four minutes until the vegetables are cooked through, but are still crunchy. If the vegetables start sticking to the pan, you will need to apply a tablespoon of water. Attach the tamari and kale, and cook for another minute.

8. Dish it with the greens and buckwheat, when the tofu is ready.

TURKEY ESCALOPE WITH SAGE, CAPERS, AND PARSLEY AND SPICED CAULIFLOWER "COUSCOUS"

Small cutlets are better, but there are two ways to turn it into an escalope if you can just locate turkey breast. You can either use a meat tenderizer, a hammer or a rolling pin to pound the steak until it's around 1/4 inch (5 mm) thick, depending on how thick the breast is. Or, if you find like the breast is too hard to deal with, and you have a strong hand, split the breast half horizontally and pound each section with the tenderizer.

SERVES 1

- 2 garlic cloves, finely chopped
- 11/2 cups (150g) cauliflower, roughly chopped
- 1/4 cup (40g) red onion, finely chopped
- 1 teaspoon finely chopped fresh ginger
- 1 Thai chili, finely chopped
- 2 teaspoons ground turmeric
- 2 tablespoons extra virgin olive oil
- 1/3 pound (150g) turkey cutlet or steak (see above)
- 1/4 cup (10g) fresh parsley, chopped
- 1/2 cup (30g) sun-dried tomatoes, finely chopped
- 1 tablespoon capers
- juice of 1/4 lemon
- 1 teaspoon dried sage

Instruction

1. Place the raw cauliflower in a food processor to produce the "couscous" Pulse to finely slice the cauliflower in two-second bursts until it resembles couscous. Alternatively, you should use a knife, then finely cut it.

2. Fry the red onion, garlic, ginger, and chilli using one tablespoon of butter until soft but not browned. Remove the cauliflower and turmeric and simmer for one minute. Remove from heat and add the sun-dried tomatoes, and half the parsley.

3. Coat the turkey escalope in the sage and a small oil, then fried in a frying pan over medium heat for five to six minutes using remaining oil, rotating regularly. Put the lemon juice, remaining parsley, capers, and one tablespoon of water to the skillet when cooked completely. That will make a cauliflower sauce to serve.

AROMATIC CHICKEN BREAST WITH KALE AND RED ONIONS AND A TOMATO AND CHILI SALSA
SERVES 1

- juice of 1/4 lemon
- 1 tablespoon extra-virgin olive oil
- 1/4 pound (120g) skinless, boneless chicken breast
- 2 teaspoons ground turmeric
- 1/3 cup (50g) buckwheat
- 1 teaspoon chopped fresh ginger
- 1/8 cup (20g) red onion, sliced
- 3/4 cup (50g) kale, chopped

For the salsa

- juice of 1/4 lemon
- 2 tablespoons (5g) parsley, finely chopped
- 1 tablespoon capers, finely chopped
- 1 Thai chili, finely chopped

- 1 medium tomato (130g)

Instruction

1. Cut the eye from the tomato to make the salsa and slice it nicely, taking care to keep as much of the fluid as possible.

2. Blend with the curry, capers, lemon juice, and parsley. You could put everything in a blender, but the end product might be a little different.

3. Heat the oven to about 220 ° C (425oF). In 1 tablespoon of turmeric, the lemon juice, and a little butter, marinate the chicken breast.

4. Put on for five to ten minutes.

5. Heat an ovenproof frying pan until hot, then apply the marinated chicken and cook on each side for about a minute or so until pale yellow, then switch to the oven for 8 to 10 minutes or until cooked (set on a baking tray if your pan is not ovenproof). Remove from the oven, cover with foil, and let cool for about 5 minutes before you start eating.

6. Meanwhile, boil the kale in a steamer for about 5 minutes. Fry the ginger and the red onions in a little oil, then add the fried kale and fry until soft but not browned for another minute.

7. Cook the buckwheat with the remaining turmeric tablespoon, as per box instructions. Serve with chicken, tomatoes, and salsa.

HARISSA BAKED TOFU WITH CAULIFLOWER "COUSCOUS"
SERVES 1

- 1 Thai chili, halved
- 3/8 cup (60g) red bell pepper
- 2 garlic cloves
- pinch of ground cumin
- about 1 tablespoon extra-virgin olive oil
- 7 ounces (200g) firm tofu
- juice of 1/4 lemon
- pinch of ground coriander
- 1/4 cup (40g) red onion, finely chopped
- 13/4 cups (200g) cauliflower, roughly chopped
- 1/2 cup (20g) parsley, chopped
- 1/2 cup (30g) sun-dried tomatoes, finely chopped
- 2 teaspoons ground turmeric
- 1 teaspoon finely chopped fresh ginger
- Heat the oven to 400°F (200°C).

Instruction

1. Slice the red pepper lengthwise around the center to make the harissa, so you have good fiat slices, cut any seeds, then put the chili and one of the garlic cloves in a roasting pan.

2. Put a little oil and the dried cumin and coriander and roast for fifteen to twenty minutes in the oven until the peppers are tender but not too hot. (Leave the oven on at this setting.) Cold, then blend with the lemon juice into a food processor until smooth.

3. Lengthwise slice the tofu and then diagonally split into

triangles each part. Put in a shallow non-stick roasting pan or one lined with parchment paper, cover with harissa, and roast for twenty minutes in the oven — the tofu would have consumed the marinade and turned dark red.

4. Place the raw cauliflower in a food processor to produce the "couscous" Pulse to finely slice the cauliflower in two-second bursts until it resembles couscous. Alternatively, you should use a knife, then finely cut it.

5. Thin out the last clove of garlic. In one tablespoon of oil, fry the garlic, red onion and ginger, until soft but not browned, then add the turmeric and cauliflower and cook for one minute.

6. Remove from heat and blend in the tomatoes and parsley, that are dried with in sunlight. Serve it with the baked tofu.

PAN-FRIED SALMON FILLET WITH CARAMELIZED ENDIVE,
ARUGULA, AND CELERY LEAF SALAD
SERVES 1

- juice of 1/4 lemon
- 1/4 cup (10g) parsley
- 1 clove garlic, roughly chopped
- 1 tablespoon capers
- 2/3 cup (100g) cherry tomatoes, halved
- 1/4 avocado, peeled, stoned, and diced
- 1 tablespoon extra-virgin olive oil
- 13/4 ounces (50g) arugula
- 1/8 cup (20g) red onion, thinly sliced
- 2 teaspoons brown sugar

- 1 x 5-ounce (150g) skinless salmon fillet
- 2 tablespoons (5g) celery leaves
- 1 head of endive, about 21/2 ounces (70g), halved lengthways
- Heat the oven to 425°F (220°C).

Instruction

1. Place the parsley, lemon juice, capers, garlic, and 2 teaspoons of oil in a food processor or mixer for dressing and blend until smooth.

2. For the salad, add the leaves of avocado, tomato, red onion, arugula, and celery.

3. Heat a frying pan on high heat. Rub the salmon in a little oil and sear for a minute or two in the hot pan to caramelize the fish surface. Transfer to a baking tray and place in the oven for five to six minutes or until it is cooked; reduce the cooking time by two minutes if you like the pink served inside of your fish.

4. Wipe the frying pan out meanwhile and put it back on a high fire. Mix the brown sugar with the remaining oil teaspoon and sprinkle it over the endive cut sides. Place the cut-sides of the endive in the hot pan and cook for two to three minutes until soft and perfectly caramelized.

5. In the sauce, mix the salad and eat with tuna, and endive.

TUSCAN BEAN STEW
SERVES 1

- 1/3 cup (50g) red onion, finely chopped
- 1 tablespoon extra-virgin olive oil
- 1/3 cup (30g) celery, trimmed and finely chopped
- 1/4 cup (30g) carrot, peeled and finely chopped
- 1 teaspoon herbes de Provence
- 1/2 Thai chili, finely chopped (optional)
- 2 garlic cloves, finely chopped
- 1/4 cup (40g) buckwheat
- 1 teaspoon tomato purée
- 1 x 14-ounce can (400g) chopped Italian tomatoes
- 1 tablespoon roughly chopped parsley
- 3/4 cup (50g) kale, roughly chopped
- 3/4 cup (130g) canned mixed beans (drained weight)
- 7/8 cup (200ml) vegetable stock

Instruction

1. Place the oil on a low medium heat in a saucepan and fry the onion, carrot, celery, garlic, chili (if used), and herbs gently until the onion is soft but not browned.

2. Mix in the stocks, tomatoes and purée tomatoes and bring to a boil. Put the beans, it requires to be cook for thirty minutes.

3. Put the kale and cook for another five to ten minutes, then apply the parsley until tender.

4. Meanwhile, according to the product instructions, cook the buckwheat, rinse, and then serve with the stew.

MISO-MARINATED BAKED COD WITH STIR-FRIED GREENS AND SESAME
SERVES 1

- 1 tablespoon mirin
- 31/2 teaspoons (20g) miso
- 1 x 7-ounce (200g) skinless cod fillet
- 1 tablespoon extra-virgin olive oil
- 2 garlic cloves, finely chopped
- 3/8 cup (40g) celery, sliced
- 1/8 cup (20g) red onion, sliced
- 1 teaspoon finely chopped fresh ginger
- 1 Thai chili, finely chopped
- 1 teaspoon sesame seeds
- 3/4 cup (50g) kale, roughly chopped
- 3/8 cup (60g) green beans
- 1/4 cup (40g) buckwheat
- 1 tablespoon tamari (or soy sauce, if you are not avoiding gluten)
- 2 tablespoons (5g) parsley, roughly chopped
- 1 teaspoon ground turmeric

Instruction

1. Mix the mirin with the miso, and one teaspoon of oil. Put the cod throughout and leave to marinate for about thirty minutes. Heat the oven to 220 ° C (425oF).

2. Heat the cod for ten minutes.

3. In the meantime, heat a large frying pan or wok with the remaining oil. Stir-fry the onion for a few minutes, then add the garlic, celery, chili, green beans, ginger, and kale.

4. Toss and fry until the kale is cooked through and tender. You will need to add a small amount of water to the pan to assist the process of cooking.

5. Cook the buckwheat exactly along with the turmeric according to the product guides.

6. To the stir-fry, add the parsley, tamari, and sesame seeds and serve with buckwheat and shrimp.

SOBA (BUCKWHEAT NOODLES) IN A MISO BROTH WITH TOFU, CELERY, AND KALE
SERVES 1

- 1 tablespoon extra-virgin olive oil
- 3 ounces (75g) soba (buckwheat noodles)
- 2 garlic cloves, finely chopped
- 1/8 cup (20g) red onion, sliced
- 13/4 tablespoons (30g) miso paste
- 11/4 cups (300ml) vegetable stock, plus a little extra, if necessary
- 1 teaspoon finely chopped fresh ginger
- 1/2 cup (50g) celery, roughly chopped
- 3/4 cup (50g) kale, roughly chopped
- 1 teaspoon tamari (optional; or soy sauce, if you are not avoiding gluten)
- 31/2 ounces (100g) firm tofu, cut into 1/4- to 1/2-inch (0.5 to 1cm) cubes (about 3/8 cup)
- 1 teaspoon sesame seeds

Instruction

1. Place the noodles in a saucepan of boiling water and cook for about five to eight minutes or as indicated on the stock.

2. For a saucepan, heat the oil; add the onions, garlic, and ginger and fry in the oil over medium heat until tender, but not browned.

3. Stir it in stock and miso and boil them.

4. Add the kale and celery to the miso broth and cook gently for about five minutes (try not to boil the miso as you destroy the flavor and make it textured grainy). As needed, you may need to add a little more stock.

5. Add the cooked noodles and seeds of sesame and allow the tofu to warm up. Serve with a little tamari in a bowl, if you wish.

CHAR-GRILLED BEEF WITH A RED WINE JUS, ONION RINGS, GARLIC KALE, AND HERB-ROASTED POTATOES SERVES 1

- 1 tablespoon extra-virgin olive oil
- 1/2 cup (100g) potatoes, peeled and cut into 3/4-inch (2cm) diced pieces
- 2 tablespoons (5g) parsley, finely chopped
- 2 ounces (50g) kale, sliced
- 1/3 cup (50g) red onion, sliced into rings
- 1 x 4- to 5-ounce (120 to 150g) beef tenderloin (about 11/2 inches or
- 2 garlic cloves, finely chopped
- 3 tablespoons (40ml) red wine
- 3.5cm thick) or sirloin steak (3/4 inch or 2cm thick)

- 1 teaspoon corn our, dissolved in 1 tablespoon water
- 1 teaspoon tomato purée
- 5/8 cup (150ml) beef stock

Instruction

1. Turn the oven to 220 ° C (425oF).

2. Put the potatoes in a boiling water saucepan, bring them back to a boil, and cook for about four to five minutes, then drain. Put one teaspoon of oil in a roasting pan and roast for thirty-five to forty minutes in the hot oven. Turn the potatoes every ten minutes to ensure cooking that everything is well cooked.

3. Remove from the oven when cooked, sprinkle with the chopped parsley and stir well.

4. Fry the onion over medium heat in 1 tablespoon of the oil for about five to seven minutes, until it is soft and caramelized. Keep on dry.

5. Heat the kale for two to three minutes, then drain. Fry the garlic gently in half teaspoon of oil for one minute, until browned but not too soft. Attach the kale and fry for another one to two minutes before tender. Keep on dry.

6. Heat a frying pan, which is ovenproof over high heat until smoking.

7. Coat the meat with half teaspoon of the oil and fry over medium-high heat in the hot skillet, depending on how you like your meat If you prefer your meat mild, it would be easier to sear it and then move it to an oven set at 425oF (220oC) for the specified periods.

8. Put it down after removing the meat from the saucepan. To pick up some meat odor, apply the wine to the hot pan. Simmer to halve the juice until it is syrupy and has a strong taste.

9. Apply the stock and tomato purée to the steak pan and bring to a boil, then apply the corn-flour paste to thicken the sauce, mix one at a time before attaining the intended consistency. Serve with the grilled carrots, onion rings, spinach, and red wine sauce and add some of the resting steak juices.

BAKED CHICKEN BREAST WITH WALNUT AND PARSLEY PESTO AND RED ONION SALAD
SERVES 1

- 1/8 cup (15g) walnuts
- 3/8 cup (15g) parsley
- 1 tablespoon extra-virgin olive oil
- 4 teaspoons (15g) Parmesan cheese, grated
- 3 tablespoons (50ml) water
- juice of 1/2 lemon
- 51/2 ounces (150g) skinless chicken breast
- 1 teaspoon red wine vinegar
- 1/8 cup (20g) red onions, finely sliced
- 11/4 ounces (35g) arugula
- 1 teaspoon balsamic vinegar
- 2/3 cup (100g) cherry tomatoes, halved

Instruction

1. To make the pesto, put the walnuts, parsley, parmesan, olive oil, half the lemon juice, and a little water in a food processor or blend until a smooth paste is in place.

2. Gradually add more water before you have the quality you want.

3. In the refrigerator, marinate the chicken breast in one tablespoon of pesto and the remaining lemon juice for 30 minutes, longer if necessary.

4. Preheat to 400oF (200oC) on a burner.

5. Heat a frying pan which is ovenproof on a high heat medium. Fry the chicken in the marinade on either side for about one minute, then put the saucepan to the oven and cook for eight minutes or until its cooked.

6. Marinate the onions for about five to ten minutes in a red wine vinegar drain gas.

7. When fried, remove the chicken from the oven, spill another tablespoon of pesto over it, and let the chicken heat melt the pesto. Cover with foil and leave for about five minutes to chill before serving.

8. Combine the balsamic vinegar with the arugula, tomatoes, and onion and drizzle. Serve with the chicken and spoon over the pesto that's remaining.

BUTTERNUT SQUASH AND DATE TAGINE WITH BUCKWHEAT
SERVES 4

- 1 red onion, finely chopped
- 3 teaspoons extra virgin olive oil
- 4 garlic cloves, finely chopped
- 1 tablespoon finely chopped fresh ginger
- 1 tablespoon ground cumin

- 2 Thai chilies, finely chopped
- 2 tablespoons ground turmeric
- 1 cinnamon stick
- 2 x 14-ounce cans (400g each) of chopped tomatoes
- 2/3 cup (100g) Medjool dates, pitted and chopped
- 1 1/4 cups (300ml) vegetable stock
- 1 1/4 cups (200g) buckwheat
- 2 1/2 cups (500g), butternut squash, peeled and cut into bite-size pieces
- 1 x 14-ounce can (400g) of chickpeas, drained and rinsed
- 1/4 cup (10g) fresh parsley, chopped
- 2 tablespoons (5g) fresh coriander, chopped

Instruction

1. Oven heat to about 400oF (200oC).

2. Measure two teaspoons of oil to fry the onion, garlic, V, and chili for about two to three minutes. Add the cumin and cinnamon and one tablespoon of the turmeric, then cook for about one to two minutes more.

3. Include the tomatoes, dates, stock, and chickpeas and gently simmer for forty-five or sixty minutes.

4. From time to time, you will need to add a little water to maintain a smooth, moist consistency to ensuring the pan doesn't run dry.

5. Put the squash in a roasting saucepan, mix with the remaining oil and roast until crispy and charred around the edges for about thirty minutes.

6. Towards the end of cooking the tagine, cook the buckwheat with the remaining tablespoon of turmeric according to the packet instructions.

7. Add the roasted squash and coriander and parsley to the tagine, and top with buckwheat.

CHICKEN AND KALE CURRY WITH BOMBAY POTATOES
SERVES 4

- 4 tablespoons extra virgin olive oil
- 4 x 41/2- to 51/2-ounce (120 to 150g) skinless, boneless chicken breasts, cut into bite-size pieces
- 2 red onions, sliced
- 3 tablespoons ground turmeric
- 3 garlic cloves, finely chopped
- 2 Thai chilies, finely chopped
- 1 tablespoon mild curry powder
- 1 tablespoon finely chopped fresh ginger
- 21/8 cups (500ml) chicken stock
- 1 x 14-ounce (400g) can chopped tomatoes
- 2 cardamom pods
- 7/8 cup (200ml) coconut milk
- 11/3 pounds (600g) russet potatoes
- 1 cinnamon stick
- 2 tablespoons (5g) coriander, chopped
- 22/3 cups (175g) kale, chopped
- 1/4 cup (10g) parsley, chopped

Instruction

1. Rub the parts of the chicken in one teaspoon of butter and one tablespoon of turmeric.

2. Leave it for about thirty minutes to marinate.

3. Fry the chicken on high temperature (the chicken should be fried with ample oil in the marinade) for about four to five minutes until it is well-browned and fried very well, then removed from the pan and put it aside.

4. Heat one spoonful of the oil on medium heat in the frying pan and add the onion, garlic, chili, and ginger. Fry for about ten minutes or until tender, then add the curry powder and another turmeric tablespoon and cook for one to two minutes.

5. Put the tomatoes to the pan and allow to cook for another two minutes.

6. Put the coconut milk, stock, cardamom, and cinnamon stick and leave for about forty-five to sixty minutes to simmer.

7. Check the pan regularly to ensure it doesn't run dry — you may need to add more stock.

8. Heat the frying pan to about 425 ° F (220 ° C). Peel the potatoes as the curry are cooking, then cut them into small chunks.

9. Place the remaining tablespoon of turmeric in boiling water, and simmer for about five minutes.

10. Dry it very well, and prepare for about ten minutes of dry steam. Round the edges, they would be soft and flaky.

11. Move it to a roasting pan, stir the remaining oil and roast until golden brown and crisp for thirty minutes. When you are through with it, put the parsley inside.

12. Add the kale, coriander, and cooked chicken when the curry has your required consistency, and cook for another five minutes to ensure the chicken is cooked very well, then serve with the potatoes.

BUCKWHEAT PANCAKES WITH STRAWBERRIES, DARK CHOCOLATE SAUCE, AND CRUSHED WALNUTS MAKES SIX TO EIGHT PANCAKES, DEPENDING ON THE SIZE
FOR THE PANCAKES

- 7/8 cup (150g) buckwheat _our
- 11/2 cups (350ml) milk
- 1 tablespoon extra-virgin olive oil, for cooking
- 1 large egg

FOR THE CHOCOLATE SAUCE

- 1/3 cup (85ml) milk
- 31/2 ounces (100g) dark chocolate (85 percent cocoa solids)
- 1 tablespoon extra-virgin olive oil
- 1 tablespoon double cream

TO SERVE

- 2 cups (400g) strawberries, hulled and chopped
- 7/8 cup (100g) walnuts, chopped

Instruction

1. Add all the ingredients together in a blender except the olive oil to make the pancake batter, and mix until you have a smooth batter. It shouldn't be too thick or too oily. (Any remaining batter can be kept in an airtight jar in your refrigerator for up to five days. Make sure to blend thoroughly until re-use.)

2. Melt the chocolate over a tray of simmering water in a heat-proof bowl to form the chocolate sauce. When warmed, mix well and whisk vigorously in the milk, then add the double cream and olive oil. You can keep the sauce warm by keeping the water in the oven, heat it to very low heat until your pancakes are ready.

3. Heat a small or medium-thick bottom frying pan before smoking starts, then apply the oil to make the pancakes.

4. Push some of the batters into the middle of the tub, then tip the excess batter around it until the entire surface is coated by it; you might need to add a little more batter to do so. If your pan is hot enough, you will just need to cook the pancake on either side for one minute.

5. Use a spatula to loosen the pancake around its edge, once you can see it go brown around the edges, then flip it over. Seek to turn over to avoid splitting it in one direction. On the other hand, cook for another minute or so, and put it in a tray.

6. Put some strawberries in the middle and roll the pancake upwards.

7. Continue doing that until you've made as many pancakes.

8. On each pancake, spoon some amount of sauce and sprinkle with some chopped walnuts.

9. Your first attempts may be too fat or fall apart, but if you find a good formula for your batter that fits better and improve your technique, you'll make it like a professional. In this scenario, preparation makes good.

SIRTFOOD PIZZA
MAKES TWO 12-INCH (30CM) PIZZAS

FOR THE PIZZA CRUST

- 1 teaspoon brown sugar
- 1 x 1/4-ounce (7g) package of dried yeast
- 11/4 cups (200g) buckwheat flour
- 11/4 cups (300ml) lukewarm water
- 1 tablespoon extra-virgin olive oil, plus a little extra for greasing
- 12/3 cups (200g) white bread _our or Tipo 00 pasta _our, plus a little extra for rolling out

FOR THE TOMATO SAUCE

- 1 garlic clove, finely chopped
- 1/2 red onion, finely chopped
- 1 teaspoon dried oregano
- 1 teaspoon extra virgin olive oil
- 2 tablespoons (5g) basil leaves
- 1 x 14-ounce (400g) can of chopped tomatoes pinch of brown sugar
- 2 tablespoons white wine

Our Favorite Toppings

1. Red onion, arugula, grated cheese (or vegan alternatives), and fried eggplant. (You can buy grilled eggplant from a local deli or market. To grill your own, heat the griddle pan until it starts smoking, then reduce the heat to medium.

2. Slice the eggplant crossways into thin slices not bigger than 1/4 inch [3 to 5 mm], spray with a little extra virgin olive oil, and barbecue until you have received black grill marks on either side of the eggplant and it's nice and crispy. Instead, roast the eggplant on a baking tray lined with a sheet of parchment paper at 400oF [200oC] for fifteen minutes or until tender and golden brown).

3. Cherry tomatoes, chili flakes, goat cheese, and arugula.

4. Red onion, rye, cooked chicken, olive and rind cheese

5. Red onion, cooked chorizo, steamed kale, and grated cheese, dissolve the leaves and sugar in the water for the flour. This will allow the yeast to become healthy. Cover with plastic wrap and wait ten to fifteen minutes.

6. Put the flours in a pot. Pair it with the dough hook if you have a stand mixer and sift the flours into the mixer pot.

7. Add the yeast mixture and oil to the flour and combine until a dough has been formed. If your dough is a little dry, you may need to add a little more fat. Knead until a soft, springy dough is covered.

8. Put the dough to an oiled bowl, cover it with a clean, humid kitchen towel, and leave it warm somewhere to rise for forty-five to sixty minutes until it is doubled.

9. Meanwhile, make the sauce with tomatoes. Fry the olive oil with the onion and garlic until smooth, then apply the dried oregano. Attach the wine and bubble to halve.

10. Add the tomatoes and sugar, put back to a boil, and simmer for 30 minutes until a thick consistency is achieved. If it's too runny, the crust can get soggy. Remove the heat from the oven. With your teeth, tear the basil leaves apart and pour them into the sauce.

11. Start kneading the dough to expel the air again — this is called knocking out, or punching hard if you have a good smooth dough after a minute or so it's finished.

12. You can either directly use the flour, or wrap it in plastic wrap and place it in the refrigerator for a few days.

13. Turn up the oven to 230oC (450oF). Dust a work surface gently with flour. Break the dough in half, roll out each slice to the appropriate size, and then put it on a pizza stone or oiled baking tray with nonstick. (This quantity of dough will make two thin-crust pizzas about 12 inches [30 cm] in diameter. If you want a deeper crust, just use more of the dough or reduce the pizza size.)

14. Spread the thin layer of tomato sauce over the dough (with this amount of dough, you'll only need about half the sauce, but freeze some left-over), leaving a space for the crust along the bottom.

15. Remove the remaining ingredients (if you use arugula and chili flakes, remove them after you have cooked the pizza). Before baking, set aside for about fifteen to twenty minutes; the dough will begin to rise again, giving it a lighter base.

16. Bake it for like ten to twelve minutes in the oven, or until the cheese turns golden brown. Now, if using, coat it with arugula and chili flakes.

CONCLUSION

———— ✐ ————

Starting up can be difficult. The plan's first week can be difficult, with days one to three reducing calorie consumption to 1000 calories comprising three drinks and one dinner. Days four to seven with an average of 1,500 calories a day are a little better. There's a whole selection of Sirtfood nutritious recipes that you can try.

In this early phase, a thinking approach is to look and feel the health effects on both your body and clothing and how your clothes match less snugly than simply concentrating on your body weight.

Feed the juices out all day long instead of getting them so close together. Take the juices at least one or two hours before and after meals, and eat no later than 7 p.m.

Although the early stage of juicing and fasting is ideal for those who might want to lose a little weight rapidly, the Sirtfood diet's overall goal is to include nutritious foods in your diet to improve your well-being and immune system. There's one more important goal, though. Although the first seven days can sound very challenging, the longer-term approach will work for everybody.

You will start the fat burning while enjoying your daily favorites by concentrating on incorporating Sirtfood rich ingredients into your everyday meals. It is an eating program and will continue to provide results for a long period.

Made in the USA
Monee, IL
21 August 2020